Intermittent Fasting 2021:

The Complete Beginners Guide to Intermittent Fasting to Rapidly Lose Weight, Burn Fat, and Heal Your Body

Felicia Renolds

Table of Contents

Introduction

Thank you for purchasing, "Intermittent Fasting 2021: The Complete Beginners Guide to Intermittent Fasting to Rapidly Lose Weight, Burn Fat, and Heal Your Body".

If you are reading this book, it is because you are interested in learning more about how you can improve your health, lose weight, boost your self-esteem and, in essence, become the best version of yourself.

As such, intermittent fasting is a wonderful option for you to achieve all of your health-related goals.

At the moment, intermittent fasting is one of the world's most popular diet plans. Nevertheless, this isn't about some fad diet, which may or may not produce results. With most fad diets, results are often unpredictable and often unrealistic. Many diets promise incredible results though they usually underdeliver.

So, intermittent fasting isn't about producing some miracle diet that will solve all of your problems. Intermittent fasting is about following solid science. This diet plan is based on a solid understanding of human DNA and evolution. Thus, we're not talking about consuming only one type of food or consuming copious amounts of another. In fact, we aren't talking about restricting your diet in any way.

What we are talking about in the intermittent fasting diet plan is about the frequency with which you eat. This is the biggest difference that you will find between this diet plan as compared to others.

The Science of Evolution

Now, when I say that the intermittent fasting diet plan is based on solid science, I am talking about the science of human evolution.

You see, humans are amazing machines that weren't built in a day. In fact, the body composition of the modern human being is the result of millions and millions of years of evolution. Therefore, it is important to understand where we, as humans, were born and where we grew up.

What exactly is the birthplace of humans is up for debate. Notwithstanding, the modern human is the result of a process of evolution which was more the product of necessity than design.

Picture for a moment, the humble beginnings of humans. Whatever belief you subscribe to in terms of the birth and evolution of human civilization, the fact of the matter is that humans had to face considerable challenges before the human race could find a foothold in the history of the world.

Early human inhabitants faced one critical issue: a lack of food.

Since early humans lacked the technology and organization that the modern human civilization currently has, early humans toiled to get any kind of food source. As such, food was scarce and forced humans to work extremely hard in order to produce enough resources to survive.

In essence, humans lived off what the land produced. It is certain that there was a steep learning curve for humans pertaining to understanding which foods were safe to eat and which weren't.

Prior to the discovery of fire, early humans had no choice but to eat fully raw fruits and vegetables. Meat products were almost certainly out of the question as there were no means for early humans to cook any foods.

With the discovery of fire, conditions began to change. Certain food could now be cooked, leading to a whole new range of possibilities in terms of dietary consumption. This new discovery enabled human society to add more food choices to the diets of individuals.

Now, these changes were gradual, to say the least. They took thousands of years to emerge and were most certainly met with fear and resistance from those individuals who were unfamiliar with the new technological advances of this early human civilization.

Fasting was the Norm for Early Humans

Since it has been clearly established by science that early humans lacked any type of reliable food source, early humans would have to go days on end before having their next meal. This led the human body to evolve in such a way that fasting was built into the genetics of the human machine.

Considering that food was scarce, especially in seasons such as winter, humans needed to build up resistance, which would enable humans to cope with small amounts of food.

This type of evolution is one of the reasons why the consumption of excess food ends up becoming stored as body fat, particularly in the abdominal area. This is due to the fact that the human body is still hardwired with the programming that was built thousands of years ago.

This storage of fat is one of the responses that the human body uses when faced with an increased amount of caloric intake. This is a very important point since the human body cannot distinguish whether you are ramping up your caloric intake as a result of a possible famine or simply because you decided to binge eat.

With the development of human civilization, food becomes more readily available. The gigantic advances made in farming and the domestication of animals led to an increasingly reliable food supply, especially when facing the harsh elements of seasons such as winter. This was particularly true of places where plants were not available year-round.

Farming essentially solves the food supply issues early human civilization faced. Farming enabled humans to produce surplus food stocks, which could be stored for those occasions in which the land did not produce, or food became scarce due to any other disruption.

Consequently, humans began changing their behavioral patterns since food production did not occupy a significant amount of their time and energy. Furthermore, the development of technology made agricultural production increasingly abundant. As a result, the human body began evolving to these new conditions.

Nevertheless, the core package of the human body is still the same as that which evolved hundreds of thousands of years ago.

Why Modern Behavioral Patterns Encourage Obesity

Since the basic package of the human body is still hardwired to survive long periods of food deprivation, the pace of modern society in which food is readily available for consumption has essentially "confused" the human body.

The issue lies in the fact that the human body is still programmed to save every calorie since the body still thinks that it may not eat again for a long time. This instinctive function leads folks to pack on the pounds as the last thing the body wants to do is give up its caloric reserves.

What does this mean?

It means that during intense periods of physical exertion, the body will actually begin burning muscle rather than fat since fat can always be transformed into usable calories in order to avoid starvation altogether.

The biological reasoning behind that is that increased muscle mass requires more and more caloric intake. So, when the body enters "starvation mode" it is prone to burn muscle, which consumes more calories, in order to save the calories it has already stored up.

This is why crash diets only work for a short while.

Starvation Mode

When a person decides to go on a crash diet, the body continues thinking it's business as usual for a given period of time. For example, if you skip breakfast or miss lunch, the body won't panic. However, if you decide to drastically reduce your caloric intake overnight, the body may think that something serious is up.

When this happens, the body may panic and enter starvation mode.

In starvation mode, the body needs to gradually shut off non-essential bodily functions in order to preserve the most important organs. This may result in a weakened immune system, decline in cognitive functions and even a halting of the body's metabolism

Since organs and bodily functions need calories in order to function, the body will save as many calories as it can in order to keep the lungs, heart and kidneys running as long as possible. Indeed, the human body is a wonderful machine.

But this wonderful machine will not be able to tell the difference between food deprivation due to a fad diet or a prolonged famine. The only thing the body is able to differentiate is the amount of caloric intake over a given period of time.

Thus, the moment the body enters starvation mode, it is virtually impossible for weight loss. In fact, the opposite may occur: the body will begin to save every calorie it can in order to ensure that it will continue functioning over an extended period of time.

As a rule of thumb, crash diets only work for a couple of weeks, at most, since the body is not designed to wait around and see if it will continue to get food. As such, the diet stops working, and the body begins to hoard calories.

Starvation mode is also very dangerous to an individual's health as decreased bodily functions, such as a weakened immune system, may lead to the emergence of health issues. These may range from a bad cold to potentially greater issues such as pernicious anemia.

How to Avoid Starvation Mode

By now, we have a much better understanding of the human body. Hence, we are able to comprehend why the body reacts the way it does in the face of certain conditions.

When you engage in intermittent fasting, you are essentially "tricking" the body to think that everything is fine despite a drastic reduction in caloric consumption.

The trick here is not to force the body to burn up its fat reserves (this is about as hard as sending people to Mars) but to help the body stimulate its metabolism so that it becomes more efficient in the way it processes foods.

The fact that modern humans have food supplies readily available means that they are eating all the time. This means that the digestive system is constantly working. And just like any part of the body which is constantly working, it gets tired and begins to slow down.

When your metabolism begins to slow down, the body has an increasingly difficult time processing food efficiently. Therefore, the usual metabolic cycle in which the body receives caloric intake processes it and excretes the leftover matter becomes slower and slower. This slower metabolic rate becomes a vicious cycle as the body becomes less and less able to process food quickly and efficiently.

Consequently, a slower metabolism leads the body to pack on more calories, the nutritious content of food is essentially wasted, and the digestive system begins to break down.

As you gain experience with the intermittent fasting diet plan, you will be able to recognize when you are genuinely hungry and when you are eating just for the sake of eating. In addition, this diet plan will enable you to get a better understanding of how your body reacts amid a significant reduction in its caloric consumption.

In future chapters, we will look into the specifics of intermittent fasting and its effects on the body. For now, I would like to highlight the fact that fasting is a much more common practice than we believe. After all, the first meal of the day is called "break-fast".

Imagine that!

This concept is already built into the language.

So, I would like to encourage you to buckle up for this ride. We are going to be addressing a number of issues related to weight gain and loss, healthy foods which you can eat on a regular basis, and which foods to avoid. This will help you get a keen understanding of how the intermittent fasting diet plan works and how you can use it to your advantage.

Also, this discussion pertaining to intermittent fasting will help you better understand the reasons why you are eating more than you should and how you can moderate your caloric intake.

Best of all, this discussion will lead you to discover the ways in which you can implement intermittent fasting as a normal part of your daily eating habits.

The time has come for you to rethink the way you approach your eating habits. By learning more about intermittent fasting and the way it can help you achieve a greater degree of health, you will be able to unlock your body's powerful mechanisms.

I am eager to get started. So, let's have a look at chapter one.

Chapter 1: What is Intermittent Fasting?

After a bit of a history lesson in the introduction, it is now time to define what intermittent fasting actually is.

We have talked about food deprivation, starvation mode and caloric intake. The fact of the matter is that intermittent fasting is more a methodology than a diet *per se*.

This is why I made the point of underscoring the difference between fad diets and intermittent fasting. Also, I highlighted the reason why crash diets almost always fail.

As such, when you understand the way the human body works, you are able to gain a keen insight into what works and what doesn't, as far as diet and nutrition plans go. This is why I have come to see the effectiveness of intermittent fasting first hand. So, what exactly is intermittent fasting?

Let's have a look at a quick definition:

In essence, intermittent fasting is a collection of various dietary methods in which the underlying philosophy revolves around the frequency of eating and not the actual consumption of foods. Consequently, intermittent fasting is somewhat of an umbrella term for these specific methods of delaying food consumption or altering the frequency with which food is consuming.

Thus, it is important to note that intermittent fasting is not about eliminating or cutting out any specific type of food, but rather, it is about determining when food will be consumed.

This dietary approach may seem counterintuitive as we have all grown up with the traditional, three-meals approach. In fact, mainstream society is built around these "three meals per day". Our lives are centered upon breakfast, then lunch, and finally dinner. Much of western culture is built on meals and food.

In fact, eating at specified times is so important that special events and occasions include eating as a part of that occasion. Sure, it is true that all cultures around the world include meals as part of special celebrations, think of a wedding for example, but western culture places special emphasis on eating. For instance, western culture places great emphasis on having dinner as a family as opposed to simply having food for the sake of eating.

When compared to other types of diets and eating plans, intermittent fasting does not restrict the consumption of any specific type of food. This is a very significant quality since most "diets" advocate for the restriction of some type of food.

This makes for diets, especially "designer" diets, unsustainable in the long run and even dangerous to your health. Many of these so-called "dietary approaches" are based on loose science and don't have any type of clinical data that can back up their claims. This is why they tend to fizzle out quickly as dieters figure out that it is not only unsustainable but does not yield the promised results. Hence, disappointment and frustration are the lingering results on dieters.

So, let's have a look at how intermittent fasting stacks up against other dietary approaches.

Crash Diets

Crash diets are popular among inexperienced dieters.

To this day, crash diets are as popular as ever since folks are still looking for quick ways to lose significant amounts of weight in the shortest period of time.

Unfortunately, crash diets only work for very short periods of time. In fact, these diets work for a few days at a time and often lead to dieters becoming undernourished and even sick. Conditions such as pernicious anemia may develop due to prolonged exposure to drastic reduction in caloric consumption.

The reason why crash diets have limited results is because these types of dietary approaches trigger "starvation mode" in the body. As I stated earlier, the body reacts to a drastic change in caloric intake by shutting down. When this happens, the body stores as many calories as possible in order to preserve essential organ function. This is why dieters quickly plateau after observing a drop in weight.

As a matter of fact, subsequent weight loss, even in starvation mode, tends to be the result of a decline in muscle mass. This is a false-positive on the results of the diet since muscle tends to weigh much more than fat. Thus, the perceived weight loss is really a change in body composition whereby the dieter loses lean muscle mass and packs on far more fat. Again, the body "panics" and begins to hoard calories.

Crash diets are also accompanied by increased physical activity. As such, the drastic reduction in caloric intake, accompanied by increased metabolic requirements as a result of increased physical exertion, is the exact recipe under which the human body evolved. The difference between modern humans and early cave dwellers lies in the fact that cave dwellers were fighting off large predators and had to forage for food, whereas modern humans engage in physical exercise for pleasure and reduce their caloric intake for dietary purposes.

Since crash diets are based on loose science and lack conclusive scientific data, it is best to stay away from these approaches and focus on dietary options which are more inclined toward approaches based on solid science.

The Zone Diet

This dietary approach has gained a considerable amount of popularity in recent years.

It is based on low carbohydrate consumption in which the dieter basically restricts their intake of carbs stemming from all sources such as flours and starches.

This dietary approach is based on the premise that carbohydrates are converted into glucose once consumed and as a result, are transformed into fat in the body only to be stored away.

In addition, this type of dietary approach emphasizes meal planning around a specific group of macronutrients which are intended to support weight loss and promote health benefits.

One such example of macronutrients are proteins. High protein consumption, in particular protein from lean meats, is intended to boost metabolism and trigger health benefits in the dieter.

However, high-protein, low-carb diets are hard to follow and require an extensive amount of meal planning and involve a very strict cooking protocol in order to ensure that the diet plan is followed per specifications.

Notwithstanding, the results offered by the Zone diet have been largely positive. Clinical research has demonstrated mixed results, which often depend on the discipline and commitment exhibited by the dieter and not so much on the approach itself. Furthermore, dieters tend to plateau in their weight loss.

One other fatal flaw of the Zone diet plan is that it is unsustainable in the long run due to the fact that this diet approach requires a large amount of planning and preparation. This can lead to trouble keeping up with the demands of the diet.

Still, the zone diet may be a viable option for those individuals who have the time and resources dedicated to keeping up with such a demanding dietary plan.

The Ketogenic Diet

The Ketogenic, or Keto, diet is another low-carb diet approach that advocates for the reduction of consumption of carbohydrates but not its total restriction.

Unlike the Zone diet in which carbohydrate consumption is completely restricted, the Keto diet is based on minimal consumption of carbs while essentially leaving the rest of the diet unchanged. Of course, the Keto diet advocates for the increased consumption of fruits and vegetables while reducing the consumption of fats and sugars. Nevertheless, its meal plans are not as restrictive as the Zone diet.

The Keto diet is based on the premise that the body's preferred fuel is glucose. As such, carbs are transformed into glucose once in the bloodstream, thus leaving fat stores untouched. As stated before, this is a natural response from the body since the body is hardwired to maintain fat stores in reserve "just in case".

As a result, depriving the body of a high amount of carbs forces the liver to produce molecules known as "ketones" from its fat stores in order to fuel bodily functions. In particular, the brain consumes high amounts of ketones as a part of its daily functions.

One very important element to note is that in order to avoid triggering "starvation mode", the dieter needs to take care and avoid a drastic reduction in caloric intake. In this manner, the body continues to believe it's business as usual, but is forced to use up its fat stores, thereby setting off a weight loss effect.

The Keto diet does call for some type of fasting though it does not fully endorse it as it is unsustainable in the long run. This point is true, especially if dieters wish to make fasting a common practice. Moreover, the traditional concept of fasting usually revolved around total food deprivation over a period of time, thus leading to adverse health effects.

On the whole, the Keto diet does have its merits and is certainly worth looking into. It pays to do your homework and certainly look into the ways the underlying philosophy and science of the Keto diet can help you achieve your weight loss and dietary goals.

Weight Watchers Program

The weight watchers program has been around for a few decades and certainly has enough data to back up its claims.

While I am not suggesting that this is the best dietary approach, it is certainly the most balanced, as it promotes healthy eating, the reduction of unhealthy fats and carbs, and advocates a moderate dietary approach aimed at promoting good health and weight loss.

Of the eating plans we have discussed thus far, the Weight Watchers program has produced the most consistent results though there is little to no scientific data that can back up its results. Notwithstanding, the Weight Watchers program is based on logic and common sense since its point system rewards the consumption of foods that are low in fat, salt and sugar, while "punishing" foods that are high in the aforementioned components.

In addition, the Weight Watchers program has gained considerable traction as several celebrities have come out endorsing the plan. Therefore, its visibility has positioned it as one of the go-to eating plans in the world.

But like all dietary plans, the Weight Watchers program is not perfect. Even though it advocates for a balanced diet based on nutritious food, dieters tend to plateau after a few weeks. This is a significant claim considering that the Weight Watchers program does not call for the elimination of carbs, or essentially any food group, but it does call for a regular food intake schedule. As such, the body learns to adapt to the foods it is consuming and end up functioning at a lower caloric-intake level. This is where the plateau effect takes place.

On the whole, the Weight Watchers program tends to be very effective, especially for those folks who have based their eating habits on high-fat, high-sugar foods and loading up on excessive carbs. This is why folks tend to see immediate results. But as I have stated, the body eventually adjusts to the new eating plan and begins to hoard calories as much as possible. As a consequence, this plateau is very hard to break, often leading dieters to "rebound" and gain weight after a certain amount of time.

How to Identify the Best Plan for You

In this chapter, we have presented the best parts of some of the most popular diet plans known today. All of these plans are based on logical assumptions, even if the science behind them is a bit sketchy. The fact remains that there is no perfect eating plan as of yet, especially since most plans go against human evolution.

Sure, there are many other plans, such as vegetarian and vegan plans, which cut out meat consumption altogether. There are also other plans which call for organic-only ingredients, and others still call for the complete elimination of carbs, sugars, alcohol and coffee in an attempt to detox the body.

All of these approaches have their merits, but they tend to be unsustainable in the long run and lead to dieters plateauing after a number of weeks. In some cases, these plans end up becoming ineffective altogether, especially if the individual has some preexisting medical condition such as hormonal imbalances, insulin resistance and food allergies such as that to gluten.

This book is not intended to hail intermittent fasting as the end-all and be-all of eating plans. Rather, it's meant to highlight the fact that intermittent fasting is based on human evolution and takes advantage of the body's natural hardwiring.

In this regard, I would encourage you to give intermittent fasting a fair chance, and I am sure you will come to see that its benefits can truly provide you with an effective alternative, especially when you have reached the plateau stage of other dietary plans.

As always, I would also encourage you to check with your doctor and/or nutrition specialist before engaging in any of these eating plans. That way, you can be sure that you will not be doing more harm than good. On the contrary, I have every intention of making sure that when you engage in intermittent fasting, you are doing what's best for you, your health and fitness goals, and that overall sense of wellbeing that comes from feeling good about yourself, both physically and mentally.

Chapter 2: Intermittent Fasting Methods

After defining what intermittent fasting is, its characteristics and how it stacks up again other popular diets and eating plans out there, the time has come to drill down and find out how intermittent fasting actually works.

As per the definition of intermittent fasting, "intermittent fasting", in itself, is not a method but an umbrella term thats encompasses the various eating plans which are based on intermittent fasting. Therefore, it is necessary to define what these methods are and how they can be put into practice in order to achieve the benefits of intermittent fasting.

What is Fasting?

When you think of "fasting", what comes to mind?

Surely, you would think about the lack of food consumption. This is the most common perception of fasting and the most generally accepted. However, "fasting" is a relative term, as fasting can range from an absolute abstention of food consumption to a more moderate approach in which fasting refers to a minimal amount of food consumption.

For the sake of this guide, the term "fasting" refers to withholding food consumption for a given period of time. That is the individual who abstains from consuming food and essentially limiting themselves to the consumption of liquids such as plain water in order to avoid dehydration.

Beyond the consumption of water, other drinks such as juices, coffee and so on are also off limits. This is very important to keep in mind since the consumption of high-sugar liquids during a fasting period will still trigger a metabolic response from the body and thereby defeating the purpose of fasting.

That being said, fasting is a lot more common than we believe.

When you have dinner and then go to bed, you enter a fasting period in which you will go for several hours without any caloric intake. Of course, this is the period in which you are sleeping. As such, your fasting period could range anywhere from 8 to 12 hours, depending on your habits and routines.

The problem for some folks may lie in the fact that these fasting periods are followed up by periods of excessive caloric intake, during waking hours, in which the individual packs on so many calories, that the digestive system and metabolism continue to work well into sleeping hours.

Based on this previous point, any version of the intermittent fasting eating plan calls for the consumption of foods that are lighter especially for dinner. This way, the body can relieve itself of having unneeded stress on the digestive system and metabolism.

Therefore, it is important that upon taking up the intermittent fasting eating plan, you begin to plan the times when you actually eat and avoid binging when you come out of the fasting period. A good rule of thumb is to eat lightly when you are coming out of the fasting period so that you don't overload your digestive system all at once.

When dieters binge after a fasting period, the body assumes that there is a lack of food and begins to store up as many calories as possible. This triggers a type of starvation mode and defeats the entire purpose of intermittent fasting.

The Purpose of Intermittent Fasting

In general, those individuals who take up any of the intermittent fasting methods do so with the aim of losing weight. While this is perfectly valid, losing weight should not be the only reason why you are looking to engage in the intermittent fasting movement.

In fact, intermittent fasting has a range of health benefits. These will be discussed at length in future chapters, but it's worth noting that intermittent fasting is not only about losing weight, but is also about provoking a reaction in the body, which can lead to improving overall health and wellness in the body.

Also, intermittent fasting creates a degree of discipline in people, which leads to losing weight and keeping it off.

That, in itself, is perhaps the biggest health benefit that can be derived from intermittent fasting: creating a healthy lifestyle in such a way that it ensures an ideal weight while benefitting from an overall improved physical condition.

That is why, at this point, I would like to encourage you to look at intermittent fasting, not just as a means of losing weight but also as means of living a healthy lifestyle that will enable you to feel good about yourself, achieve the figure you have always wanted, and ward off some diseases such as high blood pressure, diabetes and obesity. These diseases can lead to even great physical ailments such as heart disease and thereby reduce the quality of your life while increasing the probability of reducing your life expectancy.

Consequently, intermittent fasting can be your path toward a healthier lifestyle, improved quality of life and overall health benefits that you may have thought impossible to reach, in addition to losing weight, keeping it off and feeling good about yourself.

General Guidelines for Intermittent Fasting

We have established that intermittent fasting is a dietary approach which is based on withholding caloric intake for a period of time that is longer than usual.

Based on that premise, here are some general guidelines that need to be observed in order for any of the intermittent fasting methods to be effective. As such, following these guidelines will help you stay on track in the attainment of your dietary goals.

1. Consistency. This is, perhaps, the most important guideline to follow when engaging in an intermittent fasting method. By being consistent, you will be able to set a solid routine in which your body will benefit from these methods as opposed to having erratic nutritional habits, which may lead to adverse health effects. Now, there is one warning with consistency: you do need to mix things up a bit from time to time. For instance, if your choosing fasting days are

Wednesday and Saturday, your body will eventually get wise to what you are doing and lead you to plateau. Therefore, consistency pertains to following the same type of practices. In that sense, you would follow your fasting schedule on a consistent basis. So, if you decide to fast for 16 hours, it will always be 16 hours. This is not about fasting for 10 hours, and then 12, and then 20. By being erratic in your fasting patterns, what it does, is that it may trigger starvation mode in your body. That is why I encourage you to follow your fasting schedule consistently.

2. **Gradual Increments.** When you are first starting out with an intermittent fasting method, please be wary of starting out too fast, too soon. That is, be wary of suddenly fasting for 16 hours one day, especially if you have never done something like that before. Doing something like that will make your body enter into a panic and leave you sick. For instance, you are accustomed to a high-sugar diet. Suddenly, you decide to fast for 16 hours. What that will do is send a shockwave throughout your entire body and leave you reeling from the lack of sugar in your system. Eventually, you will have a drop in blood sugar that's so significant that it could land you in bed, or worse yet, in the emergency room. Therefore, I always advocate a gradual approach. So, if you haven't fasted for 16 hours in your life, you can start off by clocking in 8 hours, then 10, then 12, then 14 until you eventually reach 16. If you are going for 24 hours, then you will definitely need to work your way up to it. I compare going for full-out fasting to going from the couch to running a full marathon. While you may be able to physically endure it, you will most likely end up collapsing after a couple of miles. Since your body hasn't worked up to running such a distance, you may end up having a heart attack—literally.

3. **Balanced Expectations**. This one is a biggie. Many folks try out fad diets in hopes of dropping 20 pounds in a matter of days. Other times, folks may expect to drop 3 or 4 sizes in a week. While this is technically possible, it is neither healthy nor practical. You see, sudden weight loss may trigger the body to go into shock in order to preserve essential organ function. If you lose too much weight too soon, you might end up harming your internal organs due to deprivation. Since your body maintains a balance or at least tries to, it will panic any time that balance is upset. Think about people who have serious illnesses and lose weight very suddenly. They end up getting even sicker due to the drastic weight loss than due to the actual illness itself. So, managing balanced expectations means that you will understand that a gradual approach is, by far, more effective, and much more sustainable over the long run then dumping excessive amounts of weight in a very short period of time.

4. **Physical Exercise**. If you engage in regular physical exercise or have a profession that requires a great deal of physical exertion, then I would advise you to plan your fasting days in accordance with the demands of your physical activity. Unfortunately, it is all too common for folks who have high metabolic demands to feel dizzy, pass out, and even collapse when they are exercising during a fasting day. Since the body has been deprived of caloric intake, which it can immediately transform into energy, the body needs to transform stored fat into energy. The problem with that is, is that it takes the body a certain of time in order to do that. So, when you are exerting a great deal of physical strength, your metabolism won't be able to keep up with the requirements your body has. The end result is a very unpleasant experience which may lead to a potentially dangerous situation such as acute kidney failure.

The antidote to this point is planning fasting days in rest, or recover, days from your physical exercise. Consequently, if you go to the gym five times a week, you can choose to fast on the days which you don't go to the gym and thereby alleviate your metabolism from the increased demands of the physical exercise you engage in.

5. **Binging Right After Fasting**. This point is very important. A typical rookie mistake is having a big meal right after a fasting period. This is a terrible mistake. Since your digestive system has been on standby mode for the last few hours, it needs to slowly work its way back up to full power. So, if you decide to have a big meal right after a fasting period, you will most likely end up feeling sick.

In addition, a binge right after fasting will defeat the purpose of your fasting periods. In essence, you would be recovering all of the calories and fat that you used up during the fasting period and then some.

So, a good rule of thumb is to have something light and fresh right after a fasting period and then have a regular meal about 8 hours after you have officially come out of the fasting period. This way, you can avoid punishing your digestive system and your metabolism in one shot.

These five points are worth taking into consideration any time you are engaging in an intermittent fasting method. By following these guidelines, in addition to the guidelines outlined in each method, you can ensure all of the health benefits that come with intermittent fasting, as well as not doing any harm to your body.

So, I would encourage you to carefully plan out your fasting days so that you can have a pleasant experience and get the results you are striving for. Please bear in mind that working your way up to a full fast is necessary, especially if you haven't done it before so that you won't end up being sick at the end of your fasting period.

Chapter 3: The 16/8 Method

By now, we have established that intermittent fasting is not an eating plan in itself but an approach in which the dieter withholds food consumption for a specified period of time.

That being said, intermittent fasting comes to like through the various methods that are used in order to carry out the intermittent fasting philosophy in a practical way. As such, this chapter will focus on the first method which you can use to put intermittent fasting into practice.

This method is called the 16/8 method.

In a nutshell, this method consists of fasting for 16 hours while restricting caloric intake to an eight-hour window.

In other words, you will define a period of time in which you will consume all the food you need, thus leaving a sixteen-hour period in which you will not consume any type of food except for drinking plain water and perhaps black coffee (no sugar or cream) and tea.

Hence, the 16/8 method is a means of breaking up the fasting day, that is 24 hours, into two large blocks of time that ultimately add up to 24 hours.

This simple mathematical combination makes it easy to follow this method as it doesn't complicate things by forcing you to keep any specific schedules or force you to eat outside your usual meal times.

In addition, you are free to set the schedule that you want to follow so long as you stick to the same schedule every time you fast. This last point goes back to being consistent. When you're consistent, you are able to stick to the same procedure each time and thereby ensure that you will get the most out of this method.

In general, this method is considered to be the easiest to follow and the easiest to stick to. This is why we are covering this method first. In fact, I would encourage you to try it out before the others. Since it does not require a high degree of complexity, you can feel certain that it will help you ease into the intermittent fasting lifestyle.

Moreover, folks who follow the 16/8 method claim it produces the best results with minimum issues. Therefore, it has become the go-to intermittent fasting method, especially for those who are just starting out.

Nevertheless, I would encourage you to read in order to find out if this method is right for you. After all, you may be new to intermittent fasting or just fasting in general. Thus, the concepts outlined so far may be brand new to you and may even cause you some uncertainty about how to approach this new eating plan.

So, let's find out how the 16/8 method is composed and how you can get can started with this intermittent fasting method.

Getting Started

The first thing that jumps to mind with the 16/8 method is that it is far less restrictive than other eating plans out there. While the intermittent fasting eating plan offers a great deal of flexibility, the 16/8 method is very flexible in that you can decide when you set your eight-hour window and when you fast.

As such, the first thing you must take into account is the days per week that you will fast and the specific times that you will be withholding caloric intake.

Here are some things to keep in mind:

- Avoid fasting on days in which you have a higher level of physical exertion, such as days when you have intense workouts.
- Choose a time that does not conflict with other activities. For instance, if you choose to fast during your workday, would your fasting period interfere with your lunch hour? Would it cause some type of issue with your daily routine?
- If you are taking medication of any kind, would the times when you need to take your medication be affected by a lack of food? This is especially concerning when you are taking medication which needs to be taken with food.
- Also, take into account any conditions you may have, such as hypoglycemia, which may cause you to be sick after a given period of time without consuming food. So, you might want to avoid being away from home if you feel you might get sick.

Once you have considered these issues, you can then move on to figuring out how many days you would be willing to fast.

A good rule of thumb is picking two days out of your usual week specifically intended for fasting. These could be any two days of the week, though it is best to avoid having them be too close to each other. For instance, if you choose to fast on Mondays then fasting on Wednesdays may be too close. Perhaps you might consider fasting on Thursdays or Fridays in order to give your body a chance to recover. Over time, you can mix up the days you fast in order to keep your metabolism on its toes.

One very important recommendation is to avoid fasting on back to back days, that is, fasting for 16 hours, eating for 8, then fasting for 16 again and then going back to your normal eating habits. An approach such as this may adversely affect your body, causing you to get sick due to any number of factors such a low blood sugar or dehydration, for example.

Now, for the sake of simplicity, let's assume you have picked your fasting days like Mondays and Thursdays. These two days offer you about three days in between and perhaps don't conflict too much with your usual schedule. As such, these two days work out fine for you.

Another valuable recommendation is to avoid fasting for too many days out of the week. We have stated that a good rule of thumb would be two days, but the maximum you might want to consider is three. Beyond three days, you will be starving your body and ultimately lead to undernourishment or even pernicious anemia.

That being said, two days out of a week seem to be perfectly fine and are essentially a standard practice in the intermittent fasting community.

Now, the next step is to set your 16/8 schedule.

This implies that you will decide what hours of your fasting day you will not consume food and what hours you will be consuming food.

Generally speaking, most folks choose to set their 8-hour window during their workday. So, they may choose to eat from 10 am to 6pm. This would allow them time to have a light breakfast, a solid lunch and a sensible dinner. Then, the 16-hour fasting window would begin in which the dieter would only consume liquids such as plain water.

A schedule, such as the example provided, assumes that the individual would be at home and away from intense physical activity. Also, this assumption takes into account that the dieter would be sleeping 8 hours. So, half of the fasting period is spent sleeping.

Consequently, the fasting period begins at 6 pm and ends the following day at 10 am. This would be a great time to begin consuming food again and then carrying on with regular meal schedules.

This sample schedule basically requires the dieter to skip breakfast on the day the fasting period begins and on the day the fasting period ends. This is what makes the 16/8 plan rather easy to follow and stick to.

One very important recommendation to take into account is to avoid having a massive calorie consumption during the 8-hour window. The reason for this is that the digestive system and metabolism may become overloaded and take longer in processing the food consumed. Therefore, the real fasting period would be less than 16 hours as the body would spend some of that time trying to process the massive amounts consumed.

Furthermore, when the fasting period is over, it is highly recommended that you consume light foods such as fruit and small portions of bread, cereal and so on in order to avoid overloading the digestive system.

If you have just ended a 16-hour fasting period and you choose to go and have yourself some breakfast burritos, there is a fair chance you will end up sick to your stomach. So, in order to avoid distressing your digestive system when coming out of a fasting period, have some fruit, oatmeal, a small sandwich or some cereal, and you will be perfectly fine. By lunchtime, you can essentially have anything you want without fearing any digestive issues.

What to Eat, and not Eat, in the 16/8 Method

The 16/8 method, and the intermittent fasting approach by extension, does not call for the restriction of any specific foods. That is, the 16/8 method does not openly restrict the consumption of any specific foods. So, in theory, you could consume junk food and so on, and then enter a fasting period and then go back to your previous habits.

Unfortunately, an approach such as this would do very little to ensure the weight loss results and health benefits that would come from engaging in intermittent fasting.

This is why intermittent fasting, and the 16/8 method, call for a balanced diet that is rich in proteins, lean meats, fruits and vegetables so that the fasting periods would render the best possible results. In addition, the detoxification effects of the intermittent fasting approach would be magnified when consuming healthier foods.

Therefore, the 16/8 approach calls for a healthy diet to be combined with fasting. This is the ideal approach to be taken when engaging in the intermittent fasting eating plan.

Here is a general list of recommended foods prior to and following a fasting period:

- Vegetables (basically any type of veggie, preferably fresh, though frozen works, too)
- Fruits (the fresher the better)
- Healthy fats (the good cholesterol kind)
- Whole grains
- Lean protein (we want the proteins and not the fat)

These foods are indicative of a balanced diet that is focused on consuming protein combined with healthy fats. It's also worth noting that high carbohydrate consumption is not recommended going into and coming out of a fasting period. However, consuming carbs in moderation during regular days is fair game.

Also, great care needs to be taken in the type of beverages that are consumed. High consumption of sugary soft drinks, alcohol, sports and energy drinks may end up derailing the benefits obtained in intermittent fasting, especially if these drinks are consumed during fasting periods.

Therefore, it is vital that you not only take care of avoiding unhealthy drinks during regular food consumption periods but especially when fasting. For instance, you might be in your 16-hour window, but if you are drinking sugary sodas and sports drinks in order to remain hydrated, you wouldn't be getting the most out of the fasting period since you are still packing on considerable amounts of calories.

As such, calorie-free drinks will help curb your appetite and keep you hydrated. Black coffee and tea a good choice along with regular water. Personally, I enjoy sparkling water. It gives me the sensation that I am consuming a soft drink, but without actually doing so.

Homemade fruit juices would work well, such as freshly squeezed lemonade and orange juice. Now, in order to maintain the fasting philosophy, you would need to drink it unsweetened. Lemonade, in particular, is really good at helping you detox and avoid dehydration. So, I would encourage you to drink some during your fasting periods.

Other types of fruit juices, even if they are unsweetened, contain natural sugars. So, it would be best to avoid them altogether, though a good fruit smoothie lightly sweetened would be a great way to break out of a fasting period.

So, it pays to look into what drinks you are consuming in order to make sure you aren't packing on extra calories and sugar from drinks, especially during your fasting period.

Recommended Foods for the 16/8 Method

As I have pointed out, there aren't any specific restrictions for this method.

In essence, you can eat whatever you like. However, if you really want to get the most out of this eating plan, having a healthy and balanced diet, combined with a reduction in sugar and fat consumption will help you improve the overall effects that you will get from this dietary approach.

Here is a list of foods that are recommended for 16/8 dieters:

- Fruits: apples, oranges, peaches, all kinds of berries, pineapples
- Carbohydrates: whole grains such as brown rice and whole wheat products
- Sugar: brown sugar or molasses is ideal. It's best to avoid refined white sugar as much as possible.
- Vegetables: leafy greens are the best, also carrots, broccoli, tomatoes, cucumbers
- Proteins: poultry, fish, eggs, nuts
- Good fats: avocados, olive oil

These examples provide you with a good idea of the types of foods you should be consuming as a part of your regular diet. Nevertheless, fasting periods should be seen as a period to detox. So, if you have junk food every once in a while, the fasting period will help you get rid of these toxins. That is why you need to try your best to avoid replenishing them.

Foods to Avoid

Again, there are no specific restrictions though it's fairly clear that common sense would dictate which foods should be avoided. For example, it is a good overall practice to limit your consumption of fatty foods such as deep-fried choices or excessive amounts of sugar and carbs.

Beyond that, anything you eat outside of fasting periods is fair game. There is no need to be counting calories though having a balanced diet is more a question of good nutrition than just plain weight loss.

So, I would encourage you to limit your consumption of fat, sugar and carbohydrates. You can set up a schedule for the consumption of these foods. For instance, you can choose to have junk food once or twice a week while consuming greens every day.

What to Do on Fasting Days

When your fasting day arrives, try your best to avoid stuffing your face during your 8-hour window. Since we have already established what could happen if you eat too much in the hours leading up to a fast, I would just like to point out that a gradual reduction of caloric intake will help you ease into the fasting period.

During your eating period, try your best to consume filling foods. That way, you can curb your appetite in advance. If you eat salty foods, in particular, you will trigger the need for more food as a result of the chemical reaction in your brain.

Upon entering your fasting period, drink water when you need to. If you drink too much water, you may end up becoming dehydrated due to the loss of minerals. So, black coffee, regular tea and homemade lemonade (unsweetened) will help you get the most out of your fasting period.

Once you are arriving at the end of your fasting period, a bowl of fruit, smoothie or some other fresh fruit would make a great choice. Again, ease into your regular eating habits while making sure you have a solid meal once you have come out of your fasting period.

Benefits of the 16/8 Method

The 16/8 method certainly has its benefits:

- **Weight loss**. Current evidence supports this claim as test subjects have shown signs of losing weight due to the boost in metabolism and reduction of caloric intake. This is the main benefit of this dietary approach. Most clinical studies have shown evidence of weight loss due to fast though there is no conclusive evidence of its long-term benefits.
- **Blood sugar regulation**. Intermittent fasting has been linked to controlling blood sugar levels. Even though this type of dietary approach should be carried out by diabetics without medical supervision, most ordinary folks do exhibit a clear regulation in their blood sugar levels.
- **Increased longevity**. This is a bit of a controversial claim, but animal tests have shown that intermittent fasting does lead to increased longevity. If anything, common sense dictates that increased longevity wouldn't be out of the question.
- **Increased brain function**. The intermittent fasting approach also boosts the brain since it is forced to function on lower levels of calories. This makes the brain function more efficiently.

As you can see, the results from the 16/8 method are clear and show considerable signs of improving overall health.

Drawbacks of the 16/8 Method

Given the considerable health benefits of intermittent fasting, there are some potential drawbacks.

- **Increased eating**. This is the biggest caveat with the 16/8 method. Folks may be tempted to binge in the 8 hours prior to the fasting period figuring they will have a chance to burn off those calories. Often, they don't and end up eating more than they should.
- **Mood swings**. You may experience mood swings as a result of possible withdrawal from the reduction in sugar, fat, salt and even caffeine. So, don't be surprised if you become a little more irritable meanwhile your body becomes used to your new eating habits.
- **Physical symptoms**. Early on, you may experience fatigue, lightheadedness and dizziness. These symptoms could be the result of the reduction of caloric intake particularly if you are new to this dietary plan.

It is clear then that you need to build up gradually until you reach the full 16 hours' worth of fasting. When you manage to work your way up gradually and consistently, you will begin to notice the health benefits in a much clearer fashion.

Is the 16/8 Plan Right for You?

I would encourage you to try this method out first before you dip your toes in other intermittent fasting plans. Since it is easy to follow and does not have any restrictions, you will be able to put intermittent fasting to the test and being to see your weight loss plans come to fruition.

As always, I would also encourage you to check with your doctor before engaging in any type of diet. That way, you can be sure that whatever diet you choose to follow will be beneficial to you in both the short and long term.

So, don't be shy and give this plan a try. I am sure you will see that it's much easier to follow than most other diets.

Chapter 4: The Eat-Stop-Eat Method

In the previous chapter, we discussed the 16/8 method. We got into the depths of this method and how you can use it to implement your intermittent fasting strategy. Nevertheless, the 16/8 method is not the only one within the intermittent fasting realm.

So, this chapter will focus on the second intermittent fasting method presented in this book: the eat-stop-eat method.

The Eat-stop-eat method is simple in its approach but rather difficult in following. In essence, the Eat-stop-eat method calls for abstaining from the caloric intake for 24 hours straight.

Based on that premise, this method proves to be hard to implement since not just anyone is capable of going for 24 hours without consuming food. Indeed, this is not a method for beginners, especially if you have never fasted before in your life.

Consequently, the Eat-stop-eat method is not recommended for first-time fasters. Unlike the 16/8 method in which brand-new dieters can find an easy way to gradually ease into intermittent fasting, the Eat-stop-eat method is not exactly intended for beginners. As such, this method requires you to ease into it.

Not for Beginners

As we have stated earlier, the Eat-stop-eat method requires dieters to abstain from the caloric intake for a period of 24 consecutive hours. This does not mean that you would be having light snacks or small meals along the way. This method calls for complete abstention of any kind of caloric intake.

Consequently, the only permitted substances would be liquids such as plain water, black coffee (unsweetened, no cream) and tea (this could be any kind so long as it is not sweetened even with artificial sweeteners). It is vital that you consume plenty of water and liquids in order to avoid dehydration.

Now, if you have ever gone 24 hours without food, then you can appreciate that it is not easy to pull this off. Often, it is agony to go that long without food since our bodies become accustomed to eating at regular intervals. Since humans are creatures of habit, it is hard to break an old habit or create a new one.

This is what makes the Eat-stop-eat method tough mentally, not to mention physically. Perhaps the hardest hurdle to overcome in this method is the psychological barrier that comes with thinking that you are going to go for 24 hours without eating.

In physiological terms, it is hard enough though considering that it boils down to building habits, then it is a question of time and patience before you can ease into a full 24-hour fast. This is why it is advisable for you to begin with a less demanding method such as the 16/8 method before jumping into the Eat-stop-eat method. Once you get some experience with the 16/8 method, for example, you can jump into the Eat-stop-eat method.

In essence, you will know that you are ready to move on to a method such as the Eat-stop-eat method when you can easily pull off a 16-hour fast without feeling any difficulty in doing so. That means that you are ready to take it up a notch and move on to a 20-hour fast and then go the full 24 hours.

A Gradual, Incremental Approach

This is a point I cannot stress enough: the need for a gradual and incremental approach in which you are consistently ramping up the amount of hours you are going without food.

Now, let's assume that you can pull off a 16-hour fast without missing a beat. In that case, you can be certain that you are ready to move on to a longer fast. So, if you decided to go head first and jump into a 24-hour fast, you might find yourself feeling adverse effects of this type of fast since moving from 16 to 24 hours is not as easy as it sounds.

That is why a gradual and incremental approach would provide you with the best way for you to reap the benefits of a full 24-hour fast.

You can start off by ramping up 2-hour increments to your 16-hour fast. So, the next time you decide to fast, you can go 18 hours instead of 16. Assuming you don't feel any adverse effects, you can take it up to 20 the next time. If you still feel fine and don't feel like it's an additional drain on you, then you can take it up to 22 hours and eventually up to 24 hours.

As you can see, this gradual and incremental approach will avoid triggering a panic response from your body. This is important to keep in mind since a jump from 16 to 24 hours may lead your body to panic since it is going far longer without the caloric intake.

A word of caution: let's assume that ramping up to 18 hours poses no problem, but you felt that 20 hours was pretty taxing on your body. Then, you can stop at 20 hours for a few fasting days while your body adjusts to this long fasting period. Then, you can try to move on to 20 when you feel that you can easily handle 20.

It is very important that you monitor your body's reactions since you need to be aware of how longer fasting periods make affect your body's reactions. Since not everyone reacts the same way to similar conditions, whatever results most folks get may not apply to you in the same way.

For example, a 16 hour fast may prove to be the challenge of a lifetime to some folks but may end up being a walk in the park for you. Conversely, you may find that other folks can easily pull off a 24-hour fast but simply cannot go that far.

Whenever you are dealing with people, methods and plans are never an exact science. Different people react differently to the same things. Therefore, you must become keenly aware of how your body reacts to these changes in your fasting patterns. At the end of the day, it could be that your body simply needs more time to become adjusted to these changes as compared to others.

The Eat-Stop-Eat Method Isn't for Everyone

The difference between the 16/8 method and the Eat-stop-eat method is a full 8 hours. This is a full-time workday. As you can imagine, it is not the easiest thing to pull off. Even if you go just 8 hours between meals, you may end up famished by the time you sit down to eat again.

Therefore, intermittent fasting, generally, represents a considerable challenge to most folks. This is especially true if you have never pulled it off before.

In addition to easing into these intermittent fasting approaches in a gradual and incremental manner, it is worth analyzing if going the full 24 hours is right for you.

I would highly recommend that you try it out and see for yourself if it is really for you.

Allow me to elaborate.

The Eat-stop-eat method is preferred among athletes and individuals who have very specific targets in mind. For example, professional bodybuilders use this method during the prep stages in the weeks leading up to a competition.

The reason why a bodybuilder would resort to intermittent fasting is to keep lean muscle mass while blasting body fat. Of course, a physically demanding sport such as bodybuilding has very specific nutritional requires such as high amounts of lean proteins and carbs in order for the body to have fuel in order to withstand the often-grueling resistance training workouts.

Consequently, a bodybuilder would need to work their way up to a full 24-hour fast so that they can be sure it won't cause an adverse reaction in their body, such as dehydration, especially during an intense workout day.

Other professional athletes, such as track and field stars, do not normally engage in fasting for such extended periods of time since the demands on their bodies are quite taxing, especially due to the large amounts of cardiovascular activity. Intense anaerobic exercise requires the athlete to produce higher amounts of amino acids, for instance, thereby placing a greater demand on the caloric intake during training and competition periods.

This previous example illustrates how 24-hour fasting periods are not for everyone. So, it is up to you to determine if 24-hour fasting periods are for you. At the end of the day, the best way for you to determine if the Eat-stop-eat method is right for you is to try it out and see for yourself.

Benefits of the Eat-Stop-Eat Method

In addition to the benefits outlined in the intermittent fasting approach, the Eat-stop-eat method boasts similar benefits as the 16/8 approach.

So, why fast for 24-hours then?

Well, the benefits which you can get from the additional 8 hours' worth of fasting boil down to blasting fat and fostering lean muscle mass. This is why the Eat-stop-eat method is popular among bodybuilders since it promotes the building of lean muscle mass while reducing body fat to a minimum.

While there isn't a wealth of clinical data on the Eat-stop-eat method, there seems to be significant empirical evidence from everyday folks who claim that this method does provide effective results.

In addition, longer periods of fasting boost metabolic responses when re-entering an eating phase since it forces the digestive system and metabolism to work more efficiently in the process of foods. Therefore, it is important to consider that increasing the length of fasting periods would provide additional benefits to those seen in shorter periods of fasting.

One other important benefit from longer periods of fasting, in particular, 24 hours, is that abstaining from caloric intake will end up boosting detoxing effects in the body. Since there is no caloric intake, the body has no choice but the draw from its fast stores and continue to discharge residue from the body.

Drawbacks of the Eat-Stop-Eat Method

As with other methods, there is a downside to the Eat-stop-eat method.

This method, given that it requires dieters to go for longer periods of time without food, implies a greater demand from the body.

This is why this method is not advisable for folks who have very active lifestyles, especially if this lifestyle includes intense physical activity. This is especially important if you practice high-intensity exercises such as running or swimming.

Also, this method is not recommended for people who have specific medical conditions such as diabetes, hypoglycemia or low blood pressure. In these cases, the dieter may suffer from adverse effects, which may lead to potentially unpleasant and discomforting effects.

As such, I always advise folks who are interested in engaging in intermittent fasting to consult with their doctor, especially if they have never done anything like this before, have a preexisting condition, or are currently taking any medication.

In addition, there is a psychological barrier which may keep some folks from actually following through on a 24-hour fast. In such cases, it's best to avoid pushing yourself too far, as the potential consequences may outweigh the benefits.

Also, bear in mind that keeping a healthy and balanced diet is important as prolonged fasting periods may trigger withdrawal symptoms in folks who have a high level of sugar, alcohol and caffeine consumption. Since the body begins detoxing from many of these substances, the longer you fast, the harder the effects derived from eliminating these toxins from the body.

Therefore, it's advisable to ramp down sugar, alcohol and caffeine consumption in the days leading up to a 24-hour fast. This will ensure that you get the most out of your fasting efforts without making your time miserable.

Dietary Restrictions in the Eat-Stop-Eat Method

The Eat-stop-eat method, like the 16/8 plan, does not have any specific dietary restrictions. In addition to following a healthy and balanced diet, the Eat-stop-eat method calls for a reduced intake of saturated fats, high amounts of sugar, excessive alcohol and caffeine consumption. This would enable dieters to get the most out of the dietary plan.

This is why the intermittent fasting approach recommends having a balanced diet based around fruits, vegetables and lean proteins while limiting the consumption of foods such as junk foods, high-sugar soft drinks and excessive amounts of alcohol.

Thus, you can easily implement the types of foods we outlined in the 16/8 method, as this is essentially the same type of diet that the Eat-stop-eat method advocates you to follow. The most important thing to keep in mind is that your common sense and good judgment will lead you to make wise food choices.

What to Eat and Not to Eat Leading up to a Fasting Phase

Since the Eat-stop-eat method is rather taxing, it is important to moderate your intake of certain foods leading up to your fasting day.

Let's assume that you will begin your fast on Monday evening at 6pm after finishing dinner. Therefore, you would need to moderate your alcohol, caffeine and sugar intake throughout Monday. You may choose to drink plenty of water and fruit juices as opposed to high amounts of caffeine. Also, having a light dinner would help you transition easily into your fasting day.

Throughout your fasting day, you can consume water, moderate amounts of black coffee and tea. In addition to unsweetened fruit juice, especially lemonade, can help you stay hydrated and avoid adverse symptoms such as dizziness, lightheadedness, or even intense headaches.

So, during the day leading up to the fasting period, it would be important to have a good breakfast, a solid lunch containing a healthy dose of proteins, and a sensible dinner. This will enable your body that have enough nutrients to consume during the fasting period.

What to Eat and Not Eat after a Fasting Phase

The worst thing you can do when ending a fasting phase is to binge right after. As you gain more experience, you will recognize which foods will make you feel good as you come out of the fasting period. Try to avoid heavy meals coming out of a fasting period as you could run the risk of overloading your digestive system and consequently pay the price for it. So, I would encourage you to prepare the meals you will consume right after your fasting period.

For example, if you chose to begin the fasting period on Monday night at 6pm following a sensible dinner, you would be ready to resume eating at dinner time on Tuesday at 6pm. As such, going out for pizza or tacos may end up causing you considerable digestive stress.

So, some great options could be a hearty soup, green salad or a light sandwich such as turkey on rye. These foods will help you feel good and provide you with a filling alternative. You can then resume a normal breakfast on Wednesday morning without any restrictions.

This balanced approach would enable you to maximize the benefits of the fasting period without putting your health at risk. You can also benefit from the detoxification effects of the 24-hours while boosting the metabolic response from the fasting experience.

Considerations on the Eat-Stop-Eat Method

Just like the 16/8 method, the Eat-stop-eat method requires you to build up your stamina before attempting it. If you choose to go all-in at the outset of the intermittent fasting eating plan, you may end up causing more harm than good.

If you are new to fasting and you would like to attempt the Eat-stop-eat method, I would highly recommend that you gradually build up your way to the full 24-hour period. This would require you to make the necessary changes to your diet in order to avoid triggering withdrawal effects, especially if you have a high-sugar, high-fat diet. Also, if you consume high amounts of alcohol and caffeine, you could end up causing yourself a miserable experience.

Therefore, I would advise you to attempt a shorter period of fasting, such as 8 hours, and then beginning to ramp up the fasting period. A good rule of thumb is to ramp up 2 hours each time. So, if you start off with 8 hours, then you could move up to 10, then 12, and so on, until you are finally comfortable with reaching the 16 hours indicated in the 16/8 method.

Once you feel comfortable with a full 16-hour period, you can then continue to ramp it up. I would also like to underscore the fact that making pauses at given points in your fasting experience will help you become more comfortable with longer fasting periods.

So, if you are working your way up to a 24-hour fasting period, and you feel that 16 hours is tough, you can hold off from extending your fasting periods until you are perfectly comfortable with such periods of time.

Also, your newbie fasters, it's important to consider that getting support from those around you, such as friends and family, can help you stay on track. If you surround yourself with like-minded people, you will be able to find mental strength.

Final Thoughts on The Eat-Stop-Eat Method

Intermittent fasting is definitely not for everyone. There are folks who may not feel entirely comfortable with such prolonged periods of fasting. So, I would encourage you to give it a try before ultimately deciding if going a full day without food is the right approach for you.

Since we will be discussing one other intermittent fasting method, you will still have one more option to consider before ultimately deciding if the Eat-stop-eat method is the right method for you. Best of all, you will have all the elements you need in order to compare the methods and make an informed decision based on evidence and common sense.

After all, intermittent fasting is not a cookie-cutter approach that offers miracle solutions. So, it's important for you to figure out what works for you and what doesn't. At the end of the day, only you can decide what is the best approach that you can follow in order to achieve your nutrition and fitness goals.

Chapter 5: The 5:2 diet

In the previous two chapters, we discussed two of the most popular intermittent fasting plans. The 16/8 and Eat-stop-eat methods offer dieters two distinct fasting options in which the period in which the fasting period varies rather significantly.

In fact, the Eat-stop-eat method builds on the 16/8 method in that the 16/8 method calls for a 16-hour fasting period while the Eat-stop-eat method advocates a 24-hour period. As such, both methods are very similar though the difference lies in the amount of time the dieter is willing to go without food.

In this chapter, we will look into what is known as the 5:2 method. This method differs slightly from the previous two methods described since it does not call for the total abstention of food during any period of time, but rather, it calls for a significant reduction in caloric intake during the period of time prescribed by the method.

This is a fundamental shift in philosophy since the 5:2 method is far less restrictive in terms of the time in which the dieter will go without any type of caloric intake. Therefore, the dieter does not find themselves deprived of food but rather experiences a considerable reduction in the amount of food consumed during the fasting period.

Hence, this more practical approach has made it the most famous of the intermittent fasting methods currently available.

What is the 5:2 Method?

The 5:2 method, as described earlier, does not call to the total abstention of food. In fact, it is not a pure "fasting" approach since this method does not actually require dieters to give up food altogether during the fasting period. Consequently, the dieter is not truly fasting for any period of time.

This method was popularized by Michael Mosley, who piggybacked on the popularity of the intermittent fasting movement. This method is also known as the Fast Diet since it calls for shorter periods of reduced caloric intake as opposed to prolonged 16 and 24-hour windows.

In this method, the dieter should bear in mind that their diet should carry on as usual. Then upon the beginning of the fasting period, caloric intake should decrease to a minimum amount which would only guarantee that the individual will not go without nourishment during that window.

In some circles, the 5:2 method is considered a fad diet. While the underlying science plays off the concept of intermittent fasting, critics have singled out this eating plan as not being a real intermittent fasting method and consider it to be just another diet.

While its effectiveness has not been validated by clinical data, supporters play off the data cited for intermittent fasting, thereby justifying its effectiveness. However, this data needs to be taken with a grain of salt as most studies were done on the effects of intermittent fasting are based on the prolonged periods of fasting such as 10, 16, 20 and 24 hours. 8 hours is not generally considered as a valid fasting window since a usual person will sleep 8 hours a night. Therefore, it is too short a window to consider it to be actual fasting.

That being said, the 5:2 method does fall under the intermittent fasting umbrella and is considered to be the most widely followed plan as it does not put any significant amount of stress on dieters.

How Does the 5:2 Method Work?

The 5:2 method calls for 5 "regular" eating days and "2" fasting days; hence, the name "5:2".

When an individual engages in this intermittent fasting method, they are essentially reducing their caloric intake to a bare minimum on the preset fasting days.

Now, the fasting days can be set in the same way as they in the 16/8 and Eat-stop-eat methods. In general, dieters will choose the days which are most convenient for them. But a general rule of thumb for 5:2 dieters is to avoid weekends since weekends tend to be periods in which folks have a higher amount of caloric intake.

As such, the "regular" days are days in which there is no caloric intake restriction in any way. These are days when the individual will follow their usual eating habits and patterns. The designated fast days are characterized by a significant reduction in caloric intake. In general terms, women shall consume 500 calories while men would consume 600.

The amount of calories consumed during the fasting period have been determined by clinical data, which support a bare minimum amount of calories a person would need to consume in order to stay alive. What this means is that the dieter may virtually eat anything during the fasting window so long as it stays within the 500 to 600 calorie restriction.

In theory, a person can eat a 500-calorie hamburger and then nothing else for the rest of the fasting window. Typically, the fasting window will be a 24-hour period. Of course, having one single source of food during a 24-hour period may be stressful on the dieter and may lead to adverse effects such as those which have been outlined in previous chapters.

Thus, it is important for dieters to be aware of low-calorie foods which they can consume during the fasting window. This implies that the dieter could have three meals as per usual, except that the foods consumed would have to collectively add up 500 calories. This is important to note as it does not mean 500 calories per meal, but rather 500 calories broken up over three meals, or however many times the individual choose to eat.

Most 5:2 dieters skip breakfast on the fasting day, have a healthy lunch, and then have a very light dinner. By the time breakfast rolls around the next day, the individual may choose to have a light breakfast and then resume eating as usual.

This method is considered to be the most practical of the three we have presented herein, although it does require greater care as you would have to be sure that the foods you are consuming during the fasting period do not exceed the 500-calorie restriction. Otherwise, you would be defeating the purpose of the intermittent fasting approach.

Dietary Considerations

As with the two previous methods, there is no specific restriction on what to eat. Technically, you could eat anything your heart desires and then enter your fasting period. However, this is not recommended. As we have pointed out earlier, it is essential to have a balanced diet rich in fruits and vegetables while packing on lean proteins.

A dietary approach such as this would enable you to boost your metabolic response and foster weight loss. Then, the fasting practice would further boost your metabolic response and produce further weight loss.

As I have also pointed out earlier, having a diet heavy on sugar, caffeine, and fats may lead you to feel withdrawal symptoms during the fasting window as the body may panic at the sudden restriction of these substances.

If you are new to the intermittent fasting movements, I would highly recommend that you ease into this specific method. You could define your fasting days and gradually reduce your caloric intake until you hit the magical 500 to 600 calorie target. By the time you are able to hit your target, your body will have become accustomed to the lower level of caloric intake on specified days.

In addition, an overall balanced diet will help you prepare yourself mentally for your fasting days. As I have stated, the psychological barrier that comes with fasting can be a tough one to overcome.

So, good mental preparation is a great way of ensuring that you will stick to your intermittent fasting plans and not give up early on.

Advantages of the 5:2 Method

The 5:2 method has certain advantages, which are ideal for newbies into the intermittent fasting movement.

Since both the 16/8 and the Eat-stop-eat methods require prolonged fasting periods, newbies to the intermittent fasting movement may them intimidating and even scary. In fact, such fasting periods are the biggest objection that most folks find when considering intermittent fasting.

That is why the 5:2 method offers a rather non-threatening introduction into the world of intermittent fasting. This is due to the fact that dieters can ease into the caloric restriction and are not required to give up food altogether.

Personally, I believe this is a reasonable approach to most people, especially since the hectic pace of modern life makes it very hard to give up food altogether. This is also especially true for those folks who have intense physical exercise routines.

The 5:2 method is common with athletes across all types of sports and disciplines, particularly during training phases in which they are looking to shed weight and build muscle. This is true of athletes who play sports with a significant stamina requirement, such as soccer and basketball. These athletes will find themselves reducing their caloric intake at given points in their training so that they can keep weight off and trigger detoxing effects on the body.

For regular folks, this is a great way to boost weight loss and keep it off. Of course, bear in mind that if you consume large amounts of fat and sugar, you will find yourself packing on more weight than you would be losing. In a way, fasting periods would offset binges, thereby leaving you with no real weight loss though you may trigger the detoxing benefits of the body.

Disadvantages of the 5:2 Method

This method does not have any clear disadvantages, especially when compared to the other two methods discussed in this book.

In fact, the 5:2 method offers a very good means of introducing ordinary folks into the intermittent fasting movement.

However, there are some issues that need to be taken into consideration in order to avoid pitfalls.

Firstly, individuals need to reduce their consumption of high-fat, high-sugar foods in addition to moderating their consumption of carbohydrates. Folks who consistently consume large amounts of calories from fat, sugar and carbs may find that the 5:2 method to be very restrictive and ultimately trigger a withdrawal response from the body. So, it is worth reducing the excessive intake of the aforementioned sources.

Also, a gradual and incremental approach needs to be implemented before restricting caloric intake to bare minimum levels. Sudden reductions in caloric intake may end up doing more harm than good. That is why easing into the 5:2 is ideal, especially for those who are giving intermittent fasting a try for the first time in their lives.

It is also worth noting that you need to basically count calories in order to make sure that you adhere to the caloric restriction outlined in the 5:2 method. While you wouldn't be required to do so on a regular day, during fasting days, it is absolutely essential that you keep these calorie counts in mind.

Therefore, I would encourage you to do some research into the number of calories you would be consuming in each food during fasting days. Otherwise, you would be defeating the purpose of intermittent fasting.

Foods to Consider as Part of the 5:2 Method

We have already outlined the basics of what the 5:2 method requires in terms of foods. I would like to reiterate that there is no specific food restriction in the 5:2 method. In fact, you are free to eat whatever you wish. But as we have pointed out, it's important to follow a balanced diet in order to make sure that you get the most out of your weight loss goals.

Now, it is a different ballgame during fasting days.
During these days, you need to make sure that you are sticking to the calorie restrictions as outlined by the method. So, it's important to be fully aware of what you are eating.

As such, the first decision you need to make is how many times you will eat during fasting days. If you choose to eat three times, then each intake must take into account that you only have 500 calories. If you choose to eat twice, then you could split that up 250/250. In doing so, you would give yourself a greater amount of food, which can help you get through the day.

However, I would advise against eating just once as this will make it hard for you to get through the day. In the meantime, you can consume regular water, black coffee and unsweetened tea in order to help you feel satisfied. I also recommend unsweetened lemonade. It may taste a bit sour, but it will help you trigger weight loss and detox effects during the fasting period.

So, what can you eat during fasting days?

Here are some ideas:

- High-fiber, high-protein foods are ideal, especially lean meats and whole grains in small portions. Please stay away from carbs and starches altogether, such as pasta, white bread, potatoes, rice and so on.
- A good serving of steamed vegetables. These can be seasoned with salt and pepper.
- Non-fat yogurt with pieces of fruit and berries.
- Hard-boiled eggs with whole grain toast.
- A moderate portion of brown rice.
- Light soups such as vegetable broth, miso, or tomato.
- Drinks: black coffee, still or sparkling water and tea.

Note: please try to avoid using zero-calorie sweeteners as these generally contain chemical additives that are not conducive to the detoxing effects on your body. If you must, a natural sweetener such as Stevia may offer a viable alternative, though bear in mind that its minimal use during fasting days is ideal in order to keep health benefits.

Also, I highly recommend that you avoid eating out during fast days as you may not be sure that the food you are eating actually adheres to the caloric restriction of the 5:2 method. Thus, cooking at home would be the best way to ensure that you stick to the method.

As you gain experience in this intermittent fasting method, you will be able to develop a list of go-to foods that can help give yourself options so you can avoid becoming bored or unmotivated. So, I would encourage you to experiment until you find the right foods and alternatives for you.

What Can You Do if You Feel Sick or Uncontrollably Hungry?

If for some reason, you feel sick or just plain hungry, then you need to stop at once. You must consume wholesome food that will help get your metabolism running again. As I have mentioned earlier, there are folks with preexisting conditions such as hypoglycemia, which may trigger an adverse response in your body. When this happens, you may end up feeling terrible. That is when you must stop at once and consume some food which can regulate your blood sure.

Does that mean that it's okay to have takeout?

Well, what it means is that you should have something like which can sit well in your stomach. Then you can have a regular meal. The point behind this is that if you have a full meal when you are feeling sick, then you may end up feeling worse due to digestive distress.

The same goes if you feel uncontrollably hungry. In that case, you may choose to have something light, such as a power bar and wait for a few moments. If the feelings subside, then you might consider holding up a couple of more hours. But if you don't feel any relief, then a light meal would certainly help calm your anxiety.

The most important thing to consider at this point is that if you try to ride out these feelings, you could end up harming yourself. So, take every precaution you can in order to ensure your overall wellbeing and decrease the risk of any adverse effects.

Final Considerations on the 5:2 Intermittent Fasting Method

While this method offers a great entry-level approach to the intermittent fasting movement, it is worth noting that intermittent fasting is not for everyone.

Therefore, consider the following cases in which intermittent fasting may not be an appropriate eating plan:

- Folks who have a history of eating disorders, especially anorexia.
- Folks with preexisting conditions such as hypoglycemia, food allergies or taking medication.
- Pregnant and nursing women who have additional metabolic requirements
- People diagnosed with pernicious anemia until given medical clearance to engage in this eating plan.
- High-performance athletes who may have specific nutritional and metabolic requirements

That is why I advise folks looking into the intermittent fasting movement to consult with their doctor in order to make sure there are no medical reasons that could produce adverse effects when engaging in intermittent fasting.

Also, bear in mind that it is essential for you to make up a clear plan for your fasting days. If you do not plan your fasting days carefully, what you may end up doing is either not eating or breaking your fast by picking up any food you can find.

Thus, it certainly pays to plan ahead and make sure you always have access to the right food in order to stay on track. I would also advise you to keep a power bar stashed away with a friend, colleague or family member in case you begin to feel sick. In that case, a power bar is a quick boost of energy that will help you get through it. If the adverse symptoms persist, then you must have food at once.

Beyond these recommendations, the 5:2, in my personal opinion, is a great entry-level plan for folks who are interested in the intermittent fasting movement. This method is quite easy and can provide you with a sense of what you can expect in the 16/8 and Eat-stop-eat methods. You can then choose to engage in longer fasting periods or decide that intermittent fasting is not for you.

In any event, I always advocate having a balanced diet in which you gradually move away from high-fat, high-sugar foods so that your body can begin detoxing itself from these often-harmful substances. At the end of the day, your weight loss plans begin with simple tweaks in your regular diet.

Chapter 6: Effects on Your Body

After having discussed the three most popular intermittent fasting methods, the time has come to dig deeper into the benefits that intermittent fasting has, in general, on the body, regardless of which method is used.

As discussed at the outset of this book, intermittent fasting is an approach based on solid science and evolution in order to extract weight loss and health benefits. This approach is based on an understanding of the hundreds of thousands of years of human evolution that have led to the modern *homo sapiens* as humans are known today.

In that regard, the main purpose of intermittent fasting is to trigger the hardwiring in the body so that the evolutionary default settings kick in and produce significant changes in the metabolism and digestive system.

As we have discussed earlier, modern life has altered human eating habits in such a way that there is no longer the need to toil for food as did our ancient ancestors. This unprecedented access to food has led humans to become less and less reliant on large amounts of physical exercise in order to survive.

Nevertheless, that very access to food has made it very easy to consume ever-increasing amounts of calories. Many times, this caloric intake is unnecessary and leads to storage of calories in the body. Since the hardwiring in the body is designed to store calories in the form of body fat, any additional consumption of calories is not discarded but rather saved in the event of famine, drought or increased metabolic requirements due to increased physical activities such as running away from larger predators.

Consequently, the human body still thinks it is in a prehistoric world when in reality, it is in a completely different setting. Of course, it will take many thousands of years before the human body can adapt to the new circumstances of modern life.

So, let's jump right in and see how intermittent fasting affects your body.
We will discuss the effects in general and then hone in on positive and negative effects.

General Effects of Intermittent Fasting on Tthe Human Body

Intermittent fasting, by definition, implies a deprivation of food in the body. So, this deprivation can set off any number of reactions in the body ranging from mild discomfort to practically shutting down altogether.

That being said, it is safe to assume that intermittent fasting produces different effects on different folks. Since everyone's body is different, results and effects may vary. So, this implies that some folks may lose weight drastically while others will struggle to drop pounds. Some will find relief to preexisting conditions and illnesses, while others may find no relief whatsoever.

As such, intermittent fasting may yield different results though general assumptions can be made as to the overall effects that intermittent fasting has on the body. So, we will drill down and look at each one in a little more detail.

Detoxification

The first effect I would like to point out is detoxification.
Whether you lose weight or not, and how much weight you lose, is irrelevant inasmuch as the detoxing effect that intermittent fasting has on the body.

You see, we accumulate toxins in our bodies over time. We tend to pick them up from food, air, drinks, and basically anything we come into contact with. These toxins enter the body, and the immune system hacks away at them.

Generally speaking, the immune system will beat up toxins and rid the body of these harmful substances. However, the immune system needs certain freedom in order to function at full speed. Since the immune system is part of the overall human body machinery, it needs energy just like the other systems in the body.

Therefore, it essentially competes for energy. And when other systems in the body are overloaded, the immune system tends to become overwhelmed.

Consider this situation:
A body that is running under optimal conditions will have an immune system that is capable of fighting off just about every type of toxin. Now, let's assume there is a cold bug running around. An efficient immune system will tackle the cold bug and fight it off without causing major distress to the body as a whole.

Now, let's assume the same exercise but with a person who is experiencing serious intoxication due to the consumption of a mainly high-fat, high-sugar diet that is comprised mainly of processed and junk foods.

This person's digestive system may become so overloaded that it will take up the majority of the body's resources in order to process this food. This leaves the immune system with lesser resources to process the toxins that are derived from the food consumed. There is only so much the immune system can do, and when it is eventually overrun by the toxins, the body then begins to experience adverse reactions.

In this example, the immune system doesn't have a chance to catch up because of the constant consumption of toxic foods. The digestive system is overloaded, and the immune system is overwhelmed. This implies that the body has no choice but to begin to shut down certain functions.

In this case, these functions may be related to processing certain types of foods. Ultimately, nutrients are not absorbed properly and end up getting stashed as caloric reserves. The person ends up accumulating more calories and does not receive any of the nutrients, if any, contained in the food.

This case shows a person who is severely intoxicated and may present conditions such as fatty liver, insulin resistance or even high blood pressure. This is all due to the unhealthy diet and perhaps lack of exercise.

So, this individual decides that they will take up intermittent fasting as a means of improving their overall health.

In order to start off safe, they decide to start out with the 5:2 method.
They have analyzed which days they will fast, have planned out the foods they will consume during fasting days and gradually ease into the plan. They will begin by trimming their caloric consumption to the requisite 2000 to 2500 calories a day range in order to get a handle of reducing caloric intake.

Then, the amount of calories are reduced down to 1500, and then 1000, until reaching the 500-calorie mark. At this point, the question then begins on how to hold out an entire day on such low caloric intake.

As the individual begins to gain more stamina from fasting, they are able to go longer periods without consuming food. This will enable to body to let the digestive system clear out room, that is, process and excrete excess material in the digestive tract.

In fact, it's quite common for all of us to have matter build up in our digestive tract. This build-up leads to any number of conditions, such as a leaky gut, in which feces literally leak through the intestine and become reabsorbed by the body.

Needless to say, leaky gut is a nasty condition that leaves the sufferer's immune system overloaded by bacteria and waste matter, which shouldn't be in the bloodstream in the first place.

So, when the fasting process begins, the digestive tract begins to clear excess matter, including build up, until the digestive tract becomes clear of residue. This is part of the detoxification process. The body is now clearing waste that it doesn't need.

This process of clearing excess matter gives the immune system a chance to catch and fight off toxins as there are no new toxins coming in for a specific amount of time.

Furthermore, the body begins to build stamina since many of the body's systems are no longer overloaded. What this implies is that the body can function more efficiently since it doesn't have to compete for energy and doesn't have to deal with an overwhelming amount of work.

As the body begins to detox, the waste expelled from the organism allows organ systems to function better, the blood is improved, kidney and liver function also improves, while high blood pressure may begin to dissipate.

If this can be followed up with a balanced diet on non-fast days, then you could be setting yourself up for a dramatic turnaround, which can leave you feeling like a million bucks.

Weight Loss

The biggest reason why people engage in the intermittent fasting movement is because they are looking to lose weight.

Well, first, I'd like to point out that losing weight is not the underlying intent of people who begin with intermittent fasting. Their true intention is to look better and feel better about themselves. And that does not necessarily imply that you need to lose weight.

In fact, crash diets have a habit of forcing the body to burn muscle instead of fat. So, dieters feel that the crash diet is working, but in reality, all they are doing is changing their body composition. They are substituting lean muscle for fat. Naturally, muscle weighs more than fat. And so, the "benefits" are seen by the dieter.

But these results are not actually healthy results. They are simply a change in body composition, which in the end leads to the rebound effect among other dietary conditions.

So, weight loss needs to be taken with a grain of salt.

However, the intermittent fasting approach calls for the body to use up excess stores. This function is also improved when the individual is able to detox. So, the digestive system works much more efficiently. In turn, this kicks the metabolism into high gear giving it a chance to catch up.

When the digestive systems works more effectively, the individual's metabolism also begins to work efficiently. This makes it easier for food to be processed and expelled. If any matter should build up in between fasting days, the body will begin to discard it as it enters the fasting period.

So, the weight loss effect is essentially triggered by a combination of two phenomena: one, the detoxification of the body and, two, the improved efficiency of the digestive system and metabolism. In addition, a balanced diet that is low on fats and sugars will also aid weight loss. This becomes a formula which you can use to build a healthy lifestyle by implementing intermittent fasting as a part of your overall eating habits.

One other important aspect about weight loss: if you have a preexisting condition such as diabetes, then you may find it harder to drop some pounds and insulin resistance tends to make processing calories harder for the body. So, don't be surprised if the weight loss benefits aren't quite evident right away.

Nevertheless, empirical evidence suggests that individuals who exhibit insulin resistance but who have not yet been diagnosed with diabetes may see a dramatic turnaround as a result of intermittent fasting. This implies that the detoxification process can lead to improved levels of blood sugar and thereby alleviate insulin resistance.

Improved Blood Sugar Levels

Speaking of blood sugar levels, intermittent fasting has been linked to improving blood sugar levels. While the data on this claim is still a bit sketchy, it seems to support the fact that the lack of caloric intake, especially sugars, will enable to body to detox and begin to process intake a lot better as compared to regular eating days.

This implies that the body is able to regular blood sugar to normal levels, thereby reducing the overload that high amounts of sugar may cause on the body. In turn, this allows insulin production to level off and revert many of the adverse effects of having high blood sugar.

This regulatory effect allows the body to begin recovering its natural functions, thereby improving overall wellness. Truth be told, high blood sugar levels are a real killer since they make it very hard for the body to level out hormonal function, especially when insulin is out of whack. So, intermittent fasting is definitely an alternative for those folks who have high blood sugar levels and are looking to improve their body's overall ability to process sugar.

If you are a diabetic and taking medication, it pays to talk to your doctor about this possibility. While it may not take you off medication entirely, it may improve your dependency on medication. In some cases, empirical evidence shows folks reducing their reliance on medication to a point where they may avoid complete dependency.

So, I would encourage you to talk to your doctor in order to see if intermittent fasting can become a viable alternative as part of a holistic approach to treating diabetes and insulin resistance.

Effect on High Blood Pressure

Another interesting effect stemming from intermittent fasting is on high blood pressure.

In general, high blood pressure is associated with high levels of consumption in fat and sodium, that is, salt. When this happens, the body may trigger a reaction by elevating blood pressure in order to compensate for the constricted blood vessels.

Needless to say, high blood pressure, or hypertension, is a complicated condition that can lead to heart disease and even kidney failure. Consequently, it really pays to take care of this condition before it gets out of hand.

So, how does intermittent fasting help alleviate this condition?

Intermittent fasting, as has been stated, helps the body detox. And sodium (salt) is one of the most complex toxins in the body.

Sodium is soluble and water and is usually excreted in the urine. However, when sodium levels surpass the kidneys filtering capabilities, then one of the responses, in addition to water retention, is elevated blood pressure.

This condition will trigger the kidneys to work overtime in order to reduce the excess sodium in the body. This is where an individual may experience acute kidney failure, and if care is not taken, it may lead to chronic kidney failure.

That is why intermittent fasting is a great way in which you can clear your body of toxins such as sodium. When you restrict your caloric intake, especially if you are limiting the amount of salty foods you are consuming, then you are well on your way to giving your body a chance to catch up and eliminate a great deal of sodium in your system.

I would encourage you to drink copious amounts of water during fasting periods, even if it makes you go to the bathroom a bit often. A good rule of thumb is to drink a glass of water every 60 to 90 minutes. This will give your body enough liquid to flush out toxins such as sodium.

Of course, care needs to be taken in order not to consume too much water lest you wash away minerals and electrolytes in your urine. This condition is called hyponatremia and it basically means you have drunk too much water. So, a good rule of thumb is to stick to your 8 glasses a day, but you might consider drinking an extra glass or two in order to give your body an extra boost.

Adverse Conditions Stemming from Intermittent Fasting

We have also discussed potential adverse conditions when engaging in intermittent fasting. Aside from adverse conditions that may result from a preexisting condition such as high blood pressure, hypoglycemia or diabetes, you might run into some unpleasant symptoms due to the lack of food in your system.

The worst thing you can do, especially if you are a newbie to the intermittent fasting movement, is to go all-in on one of these methods. If you have never done any kind of fasting in your life, going all-in right away may lead you to become dizzy, fatigued, short of breath and even faint.

Therefore, a gradual approach is ideal. Earlier, we have outlined how you can ease into any of the intermittent fasting methods and thereby reduce the probability of becoming sick due to the shock it may cause your body to go all-in with any of these methods.

Now, one very important point that I would like to make is that intermittent fasting is not for everyone. There are folks who try it and find out it's simply too hard for them to go for prolonged periods without consuming food.

And, that's perfectly valid.
That is why we have included the 5:2 method, which simply calls for a considerable reduction in caloric intake but without withholding food altogether.

Of course, there are folks who simply cannot stick to an eating plan such as this one. That is perfectly fine. But just by reducing your intake of sugar, sodium and carbs can make a big difference in your overall health.

Then, there are folks who are dedicated and methodical in their approach to intermittent fasting but just don't seem to lose much weight.

The fact of the matter is that some folks may not see significant results right away. Thus, time and patience are needed before getting good results. But there are folks who start off well and then plateau. If this is your case, then you need to shake things up. Play around with your fasting schedule, maybe switch to another method, or go back to a previous one.

You see, the body is very good at adapting to changes. When that happens, the plateau effect kicks in and losing weight becomes virtually impossible. So, you need to keep this in mind when you are planning your fasting days, meals and methods.

A good rule of thumb is to shake things up every three months or so. That way, you won't give your body a chance to adjust, and you would be keeping your metabolism on its toes. So, it definitely pays to think a few moves in advance, just as if you were a crafty chess player.

As always, consult with your doctor or healthcare provider in order to make sure that engaging in any of these intermittent fasting methods is safe for you. That way, you can be sure that you will reap the benefits of your dedication to intermittent fasting and to your overall wellbeing.

Chapter 7: Intermittent Fasting and Weight Loss

Throughout this book, we have extolled the weight loss benefits which can be derived from intermittent fasting. We have established how any of the intermittent fasting methods can lead you to lose weight and keep it off. After all, the main reason why most folks engage in intermittent fasting is to lose weight and thereby feel better about themselves.

So, in this chapter, we are going to be taking a closer look at why intermittent fasting alone isn't some magic bullet that will alleviate all of your weight loss needs. Also, we will be discussing ways in which you can maximize your weight loss potential by following some simple but effective guidelines.

Cause of Weight Gain and Obesity

Since we have clearly established that the most significant benefit of intermittent fasting is weight loss, it's worth digging deeper into why you may be packing on some extra pounds or simply not succeeding at losing the weight that you want.

So, let's begin by looking at what can be causing you to pack on a few extra pounds.

First of all, your regular diet plays a critical role in holding you back in your weight loss endeavors. As we have pointed out previously, a high-fat, high sugar diet will only lead you to gain weight and have increasing difficulty in shedding those extra pounds. In addition, you might even be experiencing some health issues, as well.

Thus, the main reason why you are packing on the pounds is not so much in the amount of calories you are consuming as derived from sugar, fats and carbs, but it is the fact that your body becomes overloaded with them. This overload causes your body to fall behind and become unable to process all of these substances.

After a certain period of time, they become toxic in your body and may cause you to become intoxicated. This intoxication can become manifest in any number of ways and can cause any number of results.

For instance, you might become intoxicated with high levels of sugar in your system. So, in addition to having high blood sugar, which is a precursor to diabetes, you might end up having trouble sleeping, getting skin rashes, and even having blurry vision. These are just some of the symptoms of high levels of blood sugar.

But what having such high levels of blood sugar does to your body is cause you to become intoxicated to a point where both your digestive system and your metabolism cannot work fast enough to keep up with the influx of calories. This is especially true if you are eating all day long or if you binge. Since your body is unable to keep up, then your digestive system will find the best way to cope. In that sense, your digestive system may begin to stop breaking down foods into nutrients and send them straight to the liver.

When this happens, you begin to develop a condition known as "fatty liver". When you eventually have a fatty liver, your digestive system is essentially unable to process any foods. So, what the body does is send them straight to the fat stores.

When some folks reach this point, no matter how much they reduce their caloric intake, they still seem to gain weight. Therefore, a drastic shift in their eating habits is required in addition to medication.

This example serves to underscore the fact that your regular diet plays a vital role in determining whether or not you will be able to lose weight, period. If you engage in intermittent fasting, but you don't do much to take care of your regular diet, you may be offsetting the results you are getting from your fasting by binging afterward.

This is neither healthy nor ideal.

So, barring any physiological condition such as hyperthyroidism, your diet will play a key role in determining your chances of losing weight. However, your diet isn't just limited to the food you eat. It also refers to the drinks you consume.

Most folks don't realize that you could be consuming even more calories from drinks than you could be from food. Drinks such as sugary sodas and fruit drinks will wreak havoc on your metabolism. In addition, energy and sports drinks will do a number on your body as well. These are generally high in various types of chemicals, or they may contain artificial sweeteners, some of which, have been deemed to be unsafe for human consumption.

These sports and energy drinks may give you temporary boosts in energy and concentration but only serve to intoxicate your body. A good sign of this intoxication is when you need to consume an ever-increasing amount of these drinks in order to achieve the same results.

The same goes for alcohol.

Alcohol is very special in that the body converts alcohol into glucose in the bloodstream. When this happens, the body triggers an insulin reaction. Alcohol is processed in the liver and needs insulin in order to balance out its effect on the body.

So, when you consume large amounts of alcohol, your liver becomes overwhelmed because it is unable to keep up with the amount ingested. Since it is unable to convert it into glucose properly, the unconverted alcohol enters the bloodstream, reaches the brain and produces the drunken sensation many of you may be familiar with.

The alcohol that does get converted into glucose needs to be offset by insulin in the body. Since the body ends up being overwhelmed by the amount of alcohol in the bloodstream, the pancreas may go into shock, thereby triggering an alcohol overdose.

Granted, you would need to consume large amounts of alcohol to reach this point, but it serves to illustrate just how much alcohol can wreak havoc on your body. As such, reducing alcohol consumption to moderate levels is ideal in order to ensure proper liver function and giving your body a fighting chance to process all of your caloric intake.

Consequently, the bottom line here is that you need to moderate your intake of everything you consume in order to give your body a chance to play catch up. And by engaging in intermittent fasting, you can give your body that chance to catch up and then get ahead of the game.

A Healthy and Balanced Diet

We have indicated throughout this book that the intermittent fasting approach does not call for the restriction of any foods in any way. Technically, you could spend your regular food days eating junk food and then enter your fasting window, and then go back to eating junk food again.

While this type of approach is hardly conducive to improving your health, it is indicative of what the intermittent fasting approach enables you to do. This characteristic is both one of its biggest virtues and one of its biggest risks.

However, I personally feel that by not restricting the foods you can consume, you are giving yourself an incredible amount of freedom, freedom which must be used wisely.

That being said, the intermittent fasting approach does call for the moderation of food portions and the implementation of a balanced diet.

What does a balanced diet consist of?

Well, we have indicated that an increased amount of fruits, vegetables, lean proteins, whole grains, fiber and healthy fats are essential building blocks of a healthy lifestyle. Therefore, it is highly recommended that you begin to look at how you can begin to shift your eating habits on regular days so that you leave out much of the processed stuff and consume more of the fresh, wholesome stuff.

This requires a paradigm shift in your mindset with regard to the foods you eat and their portions.

Of course, you can still eat whatever you like, but if you limit the amount of times you eat certain foods and the size of the portions, then you are already well on your way to losing weight and keeping it off.

As such, this needs to be your starting point.

When you are able to start off by setting yourself up with a balanced diet during your regular days, then your fasting days will be turbocharged. You will kick your weight loss habits into overdrive, and the weight will begin to come off.

Best of all, if you combine a solid diet with regular exercise, you will be well on your way to creating an incredibly fit and healthy version of yourself. This will enable you to process foods better, reverse some of the adverse conditions in your body and help you regain confidence in the way you look and feel. These are just some of the ways in which you can benefit from losing weight through intermittent fasting.

But, how does intermittent fasting force your body to lose weight?

Let's take a deeper look at the science behind losing weight through engaging in intermittent fasting.

Keeping Your Metabolism on Its Toes

One of the things which I have stressed throughout this discussion is the body's ability to adapt and adjust to changes. Indeed, the human body is a marvelous machine which truly regulates itself.

However, this also means that the body is able to adapt to changes in caloric intake in such a way that the body will find the best ways to continue hoarding calories as per its hardwiring.

This is where intermittent fasting provides the opportunity to force the body to stay on its toes.

You see, as we get older, more sedentary and certainly overloading food consumption, the body packs on more and more calories. So, when you try to cut back on your consumption by reducing portions or just skipping meals, your body will quickly adapt to that and revert to its calorie-hoarding ways.

That is why intermittent fasting provides you with the opportunity to lose weight by mixing up your metabolism. What that means is that the body continues consuming calories in order to keep the body humming along on all cylinders. As long as you don't starve yourself and trigger starvation mode, the body will begin to draw on its reserves in order to the body strong.

When you fast, the body will consume whatever it has in the bloodstream, that is, the last intake of food you had prior to beginning your fasting period. When that happens, that intake eventually runs out, and the body needs to draw energy from somewhere. So, it will dip into its fat stores and convert body fat into glucose so it can be utilized as energy.

So far, so good.

You are beginning to use up body fat and make the most of your fasting period.

Things get dicey when you fast for too long and trigger starvation mode. When this happens, your body will begin to burn muscle rather than fat. This will cause you to lose weight, but rather than decreasing your percentage of body fat;s you are reducing the amount of lean muscle in your body.

Be that as it may, your is to keep your metabolism on its toes but not send it into starvation mode. So, when your body sees that the calories like before, it will accelerate its metabolism, but still maintain a business as usual attitude.

When your metabolism gets faster, what you are doing is making your body process food faster and convert nutrients into energy before it gets stored as fat in the body.

This is all solid science that has been amply proven by clinical and empirical data.

However, your body is good at adapting.

Therefore, if you fall into a routine, your body will adjust, and you will plateau. When you see that you are beginning to plateau, it's time to mix things up again.

But why wait until you actually plateau? You can take a more proactive approach and mix things up before you plateau. This will surely keep your metabolism on its toes.

Now, in order for you to mix things up, you don't need to make any drastic changes in your eating plans. All you have to do is plan for changes as you go along.

For example, you decide that your fasting days will be Monday and Thursday. After some time, this may become predictable for the body. So, you can plan to mix things up after two months and fast on Tuesdays and Saturdays.

The reason for a change such as this is that you are switching up days and the time in between those days. This makes it easy for you to plan and it makes it tough for your body to keep up. Then after the next two months, you can choose to fast on different days, or go back to the previous configuration. In any case, you are proactively giving your body the runaround.

As a final thought in this line of thought, by mixing things up continuously, you will be ensuring that your body won't get the chance to adjust and become accustomed to your new eating plan. This will help you achieve your weight loss plans and help you keep the weight off.

Mixing up Methods

One very interesting way in which you can shake things up is by mixing up your methods.

In this book, we have presented three major intermittent fasting plans which can help you to achieve your weight loss and health plans.

But what about mixing up methods?

Well, it's actually not a bad idea.

In order to illustrate this point, let's assume that we are talking about a newbie to the intermittent fasting movement who is looking to drop some pounds and just become a healthier person.

This individual little to no experience with intermittent fasting. So, it's safe to say that jumping into a 24-hour fast is essentially jumping into the deep end.

Therefore, this person can begin with the 5:2 method.

By beginning with the 5:2 method, this person can ensure that they will have a gradual introduction into fasting but without eliminating food consumption altogether. This is a great approach, especially if this person feels intimidating by the idea of going a full 24 hours without eating anything.

Since intermittent fasting isn't an exact science, this individual may take a few weeks, or even a few months, to work their way up to a 10 or 12-hour fast. For some folks, going 12 hours without food is an achievement on its own.

By this time, this individual may be inclined to give the 16/8 method a try.

As always, a gradual and incremental approach can lead this person to working their way up to a 16-hour fast. Once this individual is able to work up to a 16-hour fast, then the challenge is to keep it up until a 16-hour fast is a walk in the park.

Once this dieter feels comfortable with fasting for 16 hours, then fasting periods can be ramped up to 18, 20, 22 and eventually 24 hours.

At this point, the person can then transition into the Eat-stop-eat method. In this transition, there is an increased period of fasting which will eventually trigger all of the weight loss benefits we have outlined in this chapter.

Now, once a person is completely comfortable with fasting for 24 hours, it is not recommended to fast for longer periods of time, say, 26 or more hours. The reason for this is that you may not only trigger starvation mode, but you may even end up sending a message to your body to start shutting down organs. At that point, you might go into shock.

This last point is similar to those folks who don't sleep very much. If you have ever stayed up for 24 consecutive hours, you know how grueling it can be. If you stay awake for periods in excess of 24 consecutive hours, you may trigger a shock response in the brain, and you may simply collapse to the floor and basically enter a coma. The brain does this in order to protect the body by forcing it to sleep. It's sort of what happens to a laptop when the battery drains.

So, it is not recommended for you to fast for periods longer than 24 hours, nor is it advisable for you to have fast days too close to each other. If you attempt to do so, you might end up creating adverse effects in your body, which would end up harming you more than actually benefit you.

Of course, transitioning from a newbie in the intermittent fasting movement to mastery of a 24-hour fast is not something that happens overnight. In fact, it may take some time for you to get to that level. In fact, it may even take you a couple of years to get there. But when you eventually do, you will see a completely different version of yourself, you will feel much better about how you look, and you will certainly feel much better overall.

Final Considerations

Intermittent fasting is a great way in which you can drop weight, improve your overall health and create a lifelong plan that will help you stay in shape and keep the pounds off. This new lifestyle begins with you having a shift in your mindset in such a way that you can try to have as balanced a diet as you possibly can.

In addition, you can devise your intermittent fasting plans by choosing any one of the methods we have described herein. Perhaps you are fond of the idea of transitioning from the 5:2 to the 16/8 to the Eat-stop-eat methods.

Whichever way you choose to approach your intermittent fasting plans, you will begin to see the results in the reduction of your body fat, weight loss and overall health improvement.

So, I would encourage you to be looking at the best way in which you can turbocharge your weight loss plans and achieve the life you have always wanted to have for yourself.

Chapter 8: Intermittent Fasting and Health Benefits

In previous chapters, we have discussed how intermittent fasting can help you improve your overall health in addition to losing weight.

These health benefits have been described as improving blood sugar regulation, detoxification and improving digestive function.

However, there are some hidden health benefits that come with intermittent fasting. As such, we will discuss these hidden health benefits in this chapter so that you can see just how much intermittent fasting can help improve your overall health and quality of life. Best of all, these are practical health benefits that will seem like an added bonus to your weight loss benefits.

Increased Longevity

This may seem like a bit of a strange benefit to be derived from intermittent fasting. Now, if you really think about it, it does make sense as an overall improvement in your health will certainly have a positive effect on your longevity.

While the amount of time you live doesn't solely depend on nutrition, after all, there are numerous factors that come into play, such as genetics and environment, clinical tests in mice suggest that intermittent fasting can increase longevity.

While the jury is still out on increased longevity in humans, these tests on mice seem very promising.

Of course, it's one thing to live longer, and it's a completely different thing to live a longer and healthier life. Personally, I believe this is what we are trying to get at. It's not so much about extending your lifespan, but it's about living the best possible life that you can. So, this is a truly hidden health benefit that you can get from intermittent fasting.

Improved Cognitive Ability

The link between inappropriate eating habits, high amounts of body fat and a sedentary lifestyle with poor cognitive function has been proven across various studies.

In essence, cognitive ability, such as high-order thinking skills, such as critical thinking, are affected by a poor diet. This is the reason why undernourished children tend to fare much worse than their nourished counterparts.

In adults, cognitive ability is linked to the types of foods that are consumed in addition to rest, sleep stress and so on. In particular, having a diet high in fat and sugar promotes the oxidation of brain cells. This oxidation may also lead to plaque buildup in the brain. Eventually, plaque buildup can restrict the cognitive function to a point in which routine tasks can become a challenge for individuals.

Plaque buildup is also linked to Alzheimer's disease. Clinical studies have also pointed to the link between Alzheimer's and dementia with poor eating habits. In fact, obese adults are more prone to developing cognitive decline later in life than their fitter counterparts.

As such, intermittent fasting is a great way in which you can reduce body fat and ward off obesity. This is an example of how being physically fit can improve your overall wellbeing, in this case, your cognitive ability.

But improved cognitive ability goes much further than just reduced body fat. Remember plaque buildup?

Well, plaque buildup in the brain is a form of toxin just like caffeine, sodium, and sugar become toxins in other parts of the body. In fact, sugar has been linked as a source of plaque in the brain. Thus, there is no doubt that moderating your sugar intake is ideal for a healthy brain.

However, intermittent fasting does one very specific trick to your brain: since the brain is the organ that demands the highest amount of energy, the brain will get first dibs on all caloric intake. So, when you fast, there will be a point in which your caloric intake will end, and the body needs to draw from its reserves, in particular, to fuel the brain.

This is where intermittent fasting provides considerable health benefits.

As the brain begins to ditch plaque buildup as part of the body's detoxing process, the calorie reserves which are being burned by the body end up going to the brain. The brain is now forced to become more efficient as it does not have the same steady supply of calories as before. As a result, the brain needs to stay sharp in order to make sure it gets the job done.

There have also been some tests in which "hungry" individuals tend to do better on tests than those who are not. This is an interesting finding, and it should provide some food for thought (total pun intended). Therefore, if you are a student, intermittent fasting may help you stay sharp, especially during midterm and finals season.

Boost in Mood

Another hidden benefit of intermittent fasting is improved mood.

This is mainly due to hormonal regulation by the brain.

You see, high-sugar and high-fat diets tend to do a number on your endocrine system, that is, your hormonal balance. For instance, the pancreas is part of the endocrine system and is in charge of secreting insulin in order to regular blood sugar levels.

That being said, insulin is not the only hormone produced by the body. As a matter of fact, the body produces a host of hormones which regulate various functions throughout the body.

In this case, we are talking about endorphins or the "feel good hormones". In addition, serotonin and dopamine are all hormones that are associated with feeling good. These hormones can be triggered by exercise, having fun, engaging in loving relationships, becoming close to a higher power and so on.

However, when a person is intoxicated thanks to a diet high in sugar, fat, sodium, and so on, the brain also becomes intoxicated. Now, this intoxication is in addition to plaque buildup, which specifically affects cognitive abilities.

When the brain is intoxicated with sugar, caffeine or alcohol, there is a hormonal imbalance. This imbalance leads to a bad mood, irritability, and even anxiety. The only thing that seems to improve this bad mood is consuming ever-increasing amounts of sugar and high-fat, salty foods. In particular, chocolate has been linked to stimulating the production of "feel good" hormones in the brain.

When you engage in intermittent fasting, you are not only helping your body clear out these toxins, but you are also giving your body the chance to balance out its hormones. For instance, insulin levels will hopefully return to normal. In addition, the stress hormone "cortisol" is also reduced since the body is not intoxicated by various substances. In fact, the body orders the production of cortisol when it enters starvation mode, thereby speeding up the accumulation of fat.

When your brain is able to regulate all hormones to proper levels, you will quickly find that your mood will return to its normal state. You will feel happier and more productive as you begin to regain a better sense of who you are and how you truly feel about life.

Improved Sleeping Habits

One of the things which can absolutely trash your sanity is not being able to sleep properly.

Now, we are not talking about sleep deprivation here. That is a completely different ballgame. Sleep deprivation is when an individual can't sleep due to working long hours, military service, study habits and so on.

In this section, I am talking about problems being able to fall asleep and staying asleep. This is a form of insomnia and can be linked to intoxication in the body and the brain.

One of the many hormones produced by the brain is called "melatonin". Melatonin is the hormone that is in charge of regulating sleep cycles. For instance, the brain begins to automatically produce melatonin when the sun goes down and it starts to get dark.

On the flip side, the brain halts melatonin production when the sun comes out. This is why you often hear that the first thing you need to do in the morning when you wake up is to get some sunlight. This will automatically trigger your brain to see that it is morning and it needs to get moving.

Well, hormonal imbalances in the brain can get melatonin out of whack. This can impact your sleeping habits by reducing the brain's ability to produce enough of this hormone so that you can go to bed and fall asleep.

Also, poor melatonin production is linked to the condition in which folks fall asleep, then wake up after a couple of hours and are unable to get back to sleep. These hormonal imbalances are usually linked to abnormal levels of sugar and caffeine in the body.

Therefore, health experts recommend that you not consume caffeine for at least four hours prior to your bedtime. The same goes for consuming sugar.

As you engage in intermittent fasting, you will detox your brain from abnormally high levels of sugar, caffeine and so on while reducing plaque buildup and boosting proper hormonal balances. When melatonin gets back into its usual pattern, you will find that it is much easier to fall asleep and stay asleep.

Improved Sex Drive

Now, this might be a bit of a surprise to you, but it has everything to do with hormonal balance.

When you are highly intoxicated, and you are experiencing hormonal imbalances, all hormones become affected. And just like serotonin, melatonin and dopamine are affected, so are estrogen and testosterone.

Consequently, lower levels of production in both estrogen and testosterone may lead to a decreased sex drive. As such, it is not a psychological or physiological issue, but it is a hormonal matter. So, when you engage in intermittent fasting, your brain will regain its balance and begin to produce the right levels of all hormones.

So, in addition to improving your cognitive ability, restricting the production of cortisol, and boosting your mood through increased production of endorphins and dopamine, your body will also regulate the production of estrogen and testosterone, which could potentially lead to a healthier sex drive.

Sure, there may be psychological and emotional factors that might play into a lowered sex drive, but it certainly pays to take a look at how hormonal imbalances can affect your overall sex drive, especially if it is related to an unhealthy diet.

Of course, you might want to check with your doctor first to see if there is anything else that may be affecting this part of your life, though intermittent fasting can be a good alternative for you to improve this area of your life.

Final Thoughts

In this chapter, we covered a series of hidden health benefits that come from intermittent fasting. Most of these hidden benefits are related to the brain since the brain is the hub in which all parts of the body are coordinated.

Also, the more direct health benefits, such as weight loss, blood sugar regulation and so on, have been clearly established and are widely accepted as such despite conclusive clinical data.

By understanding how intermittent fasting can help your body improve its hormonal balance and how this can lead to improved brain function, cognitive abilities and hormone production, you are well on your way to improving your quality of life in such a way that you will be giving your body the chance to sort itself out.

Furthermore, pursuing health benefits through intermittent fasting is the ideal complement to seeking weight loss benefits. As this chapter has shown, the benefits of intermittent fasting go far beyond weight loss.

So, I would encourage you to take a closer look at these hidden benefits and see for yourself how intermittent fasting can help you achieve these benefits. After all, who wants to be miserable all the time? If you can make some tweaks to your diet and give up food every once in a while for the chance to be in a better mood all day, every day, then I believe this is a deal that I am perfectly willing to take.

I, for one, agree that intermittent fasting has helped me feel better about myself, not just by losing weight but also by being in a much better mood.

Chapter 9: Building a Healthy Lifestyle With Intermittent Fasting

By now, I am sure that you are keen on building a healthy lifestyle through intermittent fasting. I am sure that you are very much excited about the opportunities that intermittent fasting has to offer individuals such as yourself.

We have not only established the weight loss benefits that come with intermittent fasting but also the multiple health benefits that you can derive from implementing this eating plan into your life. Not only are you boosting your body's natural weight loss abilities, but you are also giving yourself a leg up in recovering your body's usual functions.

That being said, I would like to reiterate that intermittent fasting is not a fad diet or some type of magic bullet that will make you lose weight overnight, become fit in a couple of weeks and help you stay on track while you continue your old habits.

In fact, intermittent fasting is more than just an eating plan. It's a shift in your mindset which should lead you down a path to a healthier lifestyle, which you are building around one of the most important aspects of it, which is your nutrition.

As such, the intermittent fasting eating, through any of the methods that we have covered in this book, is all about finding the right balance between the foods that you love to eat and healthier options that can ensure a healthy life and a balanced diet.

But, how can you go about making this shift?

After all, we tend to fall into bad habits, bad habits that can be nearly impossible to break. It may even feel like you are pulling teeth when you think about "going healthy".

The fact of the matter is that it all starts in your mind. When you feel that you need to make these significant lifestyle changes, then you can be on your way to making them in such a way that they will be both sustainable and realistic.

I have seen folks who quit sugar, fast food and alcohol cold turkey. And what ends up happening is that they crash due to this drastic change. The change they make is so radical that their body begins to experience withdrawal, and needless to say, it is an unpleasant experience.

However, building a healthy lifestyle isn't just about eating plans; it's also about making a conscious effort to improve many different aspects of yourself.

Taking the First Step

So, how can you take the first step?

Well, I can tell you that reading this book is the first step you can take to improving your overall health and eating habits.

Even if you are a veteran of intermittent fasting, reading this book is a testament to your commitment to building a better version of yourself.

Nevertheless, you often hear folks say that they want to improve, they want to be better, yet they don't really make an effort to do so. They may try different diets and perhaps cutting back on some of their old eating habits, but the fact is that they don't really commit to making a concerted effort to improve their overall quality of life.

So, the first and biggest step that you can make is to decide to commit to a healthy lifestyle from here on in.

Now, that does mean that you are going to be counting calories, staying away from everything that is not considered "healthy" and then become a health freak?

Of course not!

Throughout this book, I have pushed the idea of a balanced diet. But a balanced diet isn't just about eating stuff that is considered "healthy". Naturally, that is a big part of it. But being healthy is so much more than cutting our sugars, carbs and other foods that don't really do much for your body.

When you cut out virtually every type of food that isn't "healthy" from your life, you are essentially making it hard for you to stay on track.

Why?

Well, the temptation is out there. Fast food places are everywhere, and junk food is cheap. Often, you are forced to make an extra effort in order to have healthy choices while fighting the urge to have something "unhealthy".

Remember the balanced diet approach?

This is where that concept fits it.

It's okay to have a burger and fries combo every so often. It's alright to have a soda, and it's certainly alright to a drink. That is why the approach that I have espoused in this book is to be moderate. If you moderate your intake of all types of foods, then your intermittent fasting efforts will have dramatic results.

How Intermittent Fasting can Really Help You Keep a Healthy Lifestyle

So, when you make a concerted effort to clean up the worst parts of your diet, you will begin to think about how you can make a healthier choice most of the time. That healthier choice will lead you to focus more on the alternatives you have rather than depriving yourself of the foods you love.

For example, you can make a healthier choice by not getting the extra-large combo at your favorite fast food place. Instead, you can think about following that up with a healthier snack later on.

Often, I have found that overeating is the result of having the option to do so. When you go to a restaurant, and they offer you the "big" menu, you often pick it, especially if the difference is only a few pennies. And then when we do get it, you might be full, but you are tempted to eat it anyway because you paid for that large menu.

By making that healthier choice, you are able to give yourself a chance to go down that healthy lifestyle path. And when you combine intermittent fasting into the mix, then you are really turbocharging your weight loss goals in addition to triggering the other health benefits that come from intermittent fasting.

At first, the biggest effect you will see from intermittent fasting is that you will begin a detoxing process. This process is critical in order for you to trigger weight loss. Bear in mind that weight will be very hard to happen if you don't detox first. The fact that your body remains intoxicated means that it will be very hard for the body to process food efficiently. Therefore, you will find yourself right where you started.

Now, detoxing can get a bit unpleasant. There might be some slight discomfort as your body sheds some toxic substances. But as you see how your body begins to eliminate toxins, you will begin to feel better about your choice to engage in intermittent fasting.

One very useful benefit to intermittent fasting is that you can "undo" a lot of the harmful substances that affect your body on a daily basis. Given the hectic pace of modern life, we don't always have the possibility of making healthy choices on a consistent basis. Thus, we end up having takeout not because we really want to, but because it's the most convenient choice at the moment.

Therefore, intermittent fasting can help reverse many of the adverse effects that come from not-so-healthy food, toxins in the environment, and stress. As such, intermittent fasting has a very powerful detox effect that can boost your body's defenses so that you can pave the way for weight loss.

As you begin to drop pounds, you will find that you will feel better, have more energy, focus and simply feel "lighter".

Over time, your body will begin to level out as you reach your ideal weight. As you approach your ideal weight, your body will begin to function all full throttle. You will see the difference in your mood, energy, focus, and well, essentially, all of the things which we have discussed throughout this book.

Tips and Strategies on Building a Healthy Lifestyle

One of the things that I have underscored throughout this book is the fact that intermittent fasting, on its own, will only get you so far. So, you need to adopt a series of positive habits which can work in tandem with intermittent fasting to help you produce the results that you want to get.

So, let's look at some tips and strategies to help you build an overall healthy lifestyle.

Getting Enough Sleep

Sleep tends to be overlooked in any healthy lifestyle plan.

A lack of sleep can do a number on your brain. One of the effects that sleep deprivation has on the body is a hormonal imbalance. As we have discussed earlier, hormonal imbalances can lead to weight gain.

In addition, sleep deprivation causes the brain to get out of whack and process food inefficiently. So, you end up eating more since the brain does not process the signal issued from your digestive system properly. So, you continue eating and eating until the brain eventually gets the "full" signal. By this time, you have already overeaten.

When your brain is working at full efficiency, it will process the signals from your digestive system more effectively, thus leading you to eat the right amount of food you need.

This is why getting enough sleep is a vital step in order to ensure that your body is running at optimum condition.

Drink Enough Water

We have also extolled the importance of drinking plenty of water.

It is a standard practice to consume plenty of water as a means of helping your body flush out toxins and other types of substances from the body. Also, drinking water is about maintaining good hydration.

In terms of intermittent fasting, drinking water is essential during fasting days. While we have made the pitfalls of drinking too much water, proper hydration is an essential part of keeping a healthy diet.

We have also made a point of cutting back on sugary drinks. It's important to keep a balanced approach when consuming drinks. This also goes for alcoholic drinks. Moderation is the key. That way, you can avoid derailing your health and fitness goals by making up the calories you are saving from food through drinking.

Of course, drinking plenty of water on regular days is also essential in order to help you continuously flushing out toxins. Thus, don't neglect drinking water. It can certainly help you stay on course.

Vitamin Supplements

Vitamin supplements are controversial as there are two schools of thought: one school supports the idea that vitamin supplements are useful and beneficial to overall health. The other school considers vitamin supplements to be unnecessary since they do not provide any additional health benefits.

Personally, I feel that vitamin supplements are useful in such cases where people actually need them. For instance, pregnant women are often prescribed additional supplements in order to ensure a healthy baby. Also, folks with certain medical conditions may need additional supplementation in order to make up for deficiencies.

In the case of regular folks who have a balanced diet, vitamin supplementation may not be needed. In that case, you would have to reconsider taking these supplements as they could even lead to vitamin toxicity. So, I would encourage you to talk to your doctor or healthcare provider in order to determine if vitamin supplementation is right for you.

Final Thoughts

Intermittent fasting is a great tool in an overall healthy lifestyle plan. When you commit yourself to making healthier choices, you can begin to turbocharge your body's natural abilities to detox, lose weight and even heal itself. Therefore, I would encourage you to take up intermittent fasting as part of a broader healthy lifestyle.

As you begin to incorporate all of these elements into your lifestyle, you will begin to gain more and more health benefits. At the end of the day, you will begin to see for yourself just how powerful intermittent fasting can be in tandem with a healthy lifestyle. Once you get on track, you will not be able to go back to your old habits. Guaranteed!

Chapter 10: What to Watch out for with Intermittent Fasting

Thus far, we have taken this opportunity to highlight the positives of intermittent fasting. We have made sure that you can see how much intermittent fasting can help you achieve your health and fitness goals.

On the whole, intermittent fasting certainly provides a great opportunity for you to lose weight and become healthier. Also, you will be able to reverse many of the negative effects that come with intoxication.

However, intermittent fasting is not perfect. There are pitfalls to consider while engaging in intermittent fasting. That way, you can be sure to watch out for these and thereby ensure that you won't fall into these traps.

So, it pays to take a closer look at each one of them so that you can get a better perspective on the potential pitfalls that come with intermittent fasting.

Willpower

The first pitfall to watch out for is willpower, that is, a lack thereof.

Most folks usually start out really motivated and committed to staying on track.

Over time, though, motivation tends to wane, especially when dieters see

that intermittent fasting is not "easy" as such. The fact that intermittent fasting is not "easy" means that there is a certain degree of discipline and willpower that is required in order to get the most out of this eating plan.

Folks who lack willpower may find it hard to stay on track. After all, going without food for an extended period of time may be a huge shock to most people. In fact, modern society extols the ease with which we can access food.

Therefore, a lack of willpower can derail your plans in a heartbeat. Of course, the worst thing that you can do is to give up. If you do choose to give up, you will be missing out on the best aspects of intermittent fasting.

Now, it's perfectly natural for you to feel overwhelmed at times. It's perfectly normal for you to feel like you don't want to go through with your fasting days or that you simply want to binge on your favorite foods.

I get all that.

We have all been there before.

But the difference between successful folks and ordinary folks is the ability to bounce back from down days. Those down days are tough, and they may become frequent over time. But your commitment to your healthy lifestyle will help you stay the course.

So, I would encourage you to build a network of like-minded folks, such as yourself, who can support you when you are down. Friends, family and partners can help you stay on track, especially on those down days when you don't feel like staying on track.

I am sure that if you surround yourself with positive people, you too will be able to find the inner strength to keep going. At the end of the day, it doesn't matter if you take a break, but the worst thing you can do is give up.

Inconsistency

Another pitfall to watch out for is inconsistency.

In order to unlock the most significant benefits of intermittent fasting, you need to be consistent. This implies that you need to be constant in your intermittent fasting methods. For instance, if you choose to fast on Mondays and Thursdays, then you need to make sure you are consistent for a few weeks as you begin to gain momentum. This will ensure that the consistency with which you fast will give your body the chance to catch up and produce the health benefits we have outlined.

A lack of consistency is the type of situation which can adversely affect your health and fitness objectives since the end result may be a lack of weight loss, persistent symptoms and other negative health condition which may simply not go away.

In this regard, being consistent is the right way for you to give your body the chance to catch up, detox and produce the health benefits you have set for yourself.

Think of it this way:

You need money in order to pay the bills. Now, you have gotten a job in which you only go once a week. Since you are paid per hour, you will only get paid for the hours you work.

Now, let's assume that you need $100 to pay all of your bills. Your hourly wage is $5 an hour. As such, you would need to work 20 hours in order to get the $100 you need to pay your bills. If you worked for 8 hours a day, you would have the $100 you need after 3 full days of work. But if you only went to work once a week, then you would need three weeks in order to get the $100 you need.

Of course, working once a week is a lot more comfortable than working from Monday to Friday, but you will not be able to meet your financial goals.

Well, intermittent fasting works exactly the same way.
If you decide to fast one week and then skip three weeks at a time without making any significant changes in your lifestyle, then you are doing yourself a great disservice. By being inconsistent, you are not giving your body the chance to ease into a new dietary paradigm, which can boost the better parts of your biology.

If anything, you might trigger a shock reaction in your body by suddenly withholding food on a random day. Your body may take it as a sign of an unexpected event and may begin to shut down in order to protect itself from harm.

So, I would greatly encourage you to be as consistent as you can. Of course, skipping a day here and there will do no harm to your fasting regimen. But please try to stay on course as much as you can. This will ensure that you will get the benefits we have outlined throughout this book.

Doing Intermittent Fasting Without any Lifestyle Changes

There are folks who may decide to engage in intermittent fasting without making any substantial lifestyle changes thinking that intermittent fasting will detox them from everything they consume on a regular basis.

Now, I would say that that is better than nothing. But it is not as effective as if you made significant lifestyle changes.

When you continue with unhealthy lifestyle habits, you are pumping your body full of harmful substances which will not be entirely eliminated through intermittent fasting. In fact, you may trigger a withdrawal response from your body by suddenly cutting off substances such as sugar and caffeine.

By doing this, the last thing you will see is weight loss or health benefits. Instead, you will end up going through unpleasant experiences every time you attempt to fast.

In the end, this type of approach leads folks to dismiss intermittent fasting by saying that it is ineffective when in reality, they didn't set themselves up for success. They went about the approach in the wrong way and thereby hindered their chances of losing weight and achieving the most important health benefits that stem from intermittent fasting.

So, I would encourage you to set yourself up for success by gradually making the lifestyle changes that you feel would best suit your health and fitness needs.

Perhaps you have an overall balanced lifestyle but drink too much coffee. Then, you can make a plan to reduce your caffeine intake. Or, you might be eating too much sugar and dairy. So, you could make a plan to gradually cut down on these foods. The idea is not to cut them out completely, but rather, just cut back on them so that you can give your body the chance to process everything still in the system and, in essence, start over fresh.

Unrealistic Expectations

For some folks, losing weight is a constant challenge throughout their lives. There are folks who struggle with keeping weight off and seemingly gain weight by just thinking about food.

If you have struggled with weight over the course of your life, you may have come to find intermittent fasting as a potential option for you to address your weight issues. I can assure you that, if done properly, you will find a viable alternative to losing weight.

The problem may be with your expectations. In modern life, we are all looking to get instant results. The fact that modern technology has enabled instant communications and instant gratification, we often tend to see a lack of immediate results as a failure.

However, losing weight has never been a short-term proposition.

Sure, there are times when you can lose a good deal of weight in a short period of time. But, losing a great deal of weight in a short period of time is both unhealthy and impractical.

If you lose a great deal of weight in a very short period of time, say 20 pounds a week, your body will go into shock. Since the body doesn't understand why you are losing so much weight, it will think that something is wrong and begin to shut down in order to protect internal organs and vital systems functions.

If you keep realistic expectations, you will be able to give yourself the time you need in order to see real results. It may take you some weeks before you start to notice a difference but rest assured that if you are consistent, you will begin to see the results you want soon enough.

In a way, it's like investing in a business. You shouldn't expect to see profits on the first day you open a new business. But if you manage it right, you will soon begin to see the benefits of running a successful business in the income it is able to produce.

Intermittent fasting works the same way. There is a lag between the beginning of fasting and the time when you begin to see results.

Consequently, don't become discouraged if you don't see results right away. Give it a fair chance, and you will soon see the benefits of this approach. As I have stated, the worst thing you can do is give up.

Unfair Comparisons

The last pitfall I would like to warn you about is unfair comparisons.

If you have done your homework on intermittent fasting, I am sure you have seen websites, books and experts claiming that they lost "X" amount of weight in "Y" amount of time. They have lost unbelievable amounts of weight in a short period of time.

However, these types of claims need to be taken with a grain of salt. While it is true that many people have achieved remarkable results from intermittent fasting, some of those success stories you read about may just be a bunch of baloney used to sell books.

This is where unfair comparisons are born. You see that one individual has achieved a certain result. And while it may be true that they really were able to achieve those results, it would be unfair to you to compare yourself to them.

Bear in mind that all bodies are different, and all people have different rhythms. You may have a naturally faster metabolism than other folks, and so you may be able to get better results sooner. Perhaps you have a slower metabolism, and so you don't get the same results as the next person.

As long as you are on track and you see the benefits, don't fall prey to comparing yourself to other folks. You are only setting yourself up for trouble by comparing yourself to other folks. Sure, you can try and learn from them, see what has made them successful, but at the end of the day, if you don't have the same results as they do, don't beat yourself up over time.

By being consistent and making lifestyle changes, you will be able to set yourself up for success. Then, the only person you need to compare your results with is yourself. As long as you can see that you have been successful, then what everyone else does becomes secondary.

Chapter 11: Safety and Side Effects to Consider with Intermittent Fasting

The last chapter in this book is dedicated to providing some words of caution about how intermittent fasting may adversely affect you and what you need to look out for in case something isn't right.

In addition, this chapter will discuss circumstances under which some folks should proceed with caution when attempting intermittent fasting.

First, we will focus on a side effect that may arise from intermittent fasting. These side effects may result from the reaction the body will get from withholding certain substances from the body. So, it pays to keep an eye out for some of these symptoms before they develop into something potentially serious.

Withdrawal

I have referred to withdrawal on several occasions throughout this book.

In essence, withdrawal is triggered when the body lacks a substance to which it has, essentially, become addicted.

When most people think of withdrawal, they tend to think about drug abuse and alcohol. Sure, these are the most extremes examples of that. It is common to see drug addicts and alcoholics have violent reactions during detox periods. These reactions are not just unpleasant but may even put their life at risk.

Now, I am not suggesting that you will go into this type of withdrawal, but an abrupt elimination of substances such as caffeine and sugar can trigger some mild reactions such as headaches and dizziness, to some more brutal reactions like low blood pressure and even fainting. In addition, withdrawal is accompanied by irritability and an overall sense of discomfort.

In a way, withdrawal is positive as it is a sign that your body is ridding itself of this toxic substance. However, the process is unpleasant and may lead to some of the reactions we have discussed. As such, there is no need to go through this experience if you are able to gradually cut back from these substances.

If you are experiencing withdrawal symptoms, I would urge you to seek medical attention at once. These symptoms, if left unattended, may cause you to faint while operating a vehicle or lose consciousness momentarily. So, it's best to nip things in the bud in case you feel you cannot deal with these symptoms.

Anxiety Attacks

Another potential side effect of detoxing through intermittent fasting is the potential for an anxiety attack. This can happen when you are withholding food for an extended period of time, especially if you are new to intermittent fasting.

An anxiety attack may come upon you because you feel that you are not getting enough nutrition, or you are missing your usual feeding times. For instance, there are folks who eat once every 30 minutes. So, if you go 2 or 3 hours without eating, you may begin to feel anxious. The anxiety may begin to rise when you realize that it will still be a few more hours before you can eat again.

In this case, anxiety may set in as shortness of breath, a feeling of desperation and just a general sensation of panic.

I would say that it's perfectly natural for someone who is new to intermittent fasting to feel some sort of anxiety and overall uneasiness about what to expect. However, when these feelings get out of hand, it's just best to have something to eat and drink. It could be something simple as a cup of coffee and a low-fat muffin. But the main point is to receive nourishment as soon as possible. When you feel that the anxiety begins to subside, then you can either resume your fasting period, that is, attempt to carry on as planned, or stop at once and eat at the next meal time.

The one thing that I would like to warn you about is to avoid binging when you feel anxiety setting in as you could really harm yourself by eating way too much after withholding food for any length of time.

Digestive Distress

Since intermittent fasting has a detoxing component to it, you may experience digestive distress during your first few experiences. This is due to your body flushing out much of the residual matter in your body in addition to simply excreting whatever is still left over in the digestive tract.

While this is normal to a certain extent, care should be taken if you happen to experience severe diarrhea. This may be especially true if you jump into a fasting period after overeating the previous day. As long as it isn't anything that you feel to be abnormal, then you can attribute it to the detoxing process. However, if symptoms do not subside, then you may need to seek medical attention at once.

Another symptom of digestive distress is discomfort, pain and cramps. This may happen in case you haven't tried fasting before, and you are new to it. You may also experience this type of symptoms when you are extending your fasting periods. For example, you are going from 8 hours to, say, 12 hours.

These symptoms may occur as stomach acids may irritate the walls of the stomach. In which case, you may need to have some type of food in order to give your stomach acids something to work on. If the pain is severe, then you may need to seek medical attention as it could be a sign of a digestive condition such as Irritable Bowel Syndrome or even an ulcer. At the end of the day, your doctor will determine if there is actually something wrong that needs to be addressed.

Headaches

One other symptom that may affect you during fasting is a headache. This is a natural reaction by the brain to the sudden change in chemical composition as a result of the detoxing process. You may find that you get a slight headache that will go away on its own.

However, a strong headache and persistent headache may be a side effect of the detoxing process or just a lack of food. Since you have an empty stomach, taking headache medication would be ill-advised as it may trigger digestive distress. If your headache is unbearable, then you may need to have food with the medication.

Regular painkillers such as Aspirin and Tylenol don't normally cause adverse effects on your stomach, but given the fasting period, it would be best for you to have some food with the medication. That way, you can find comfort and relief. Again, if the symptoms persist and are too strong for you to cope, then please seek medical attention at once.

Preexisting Conditions

Another of the cautions we have issued in this book is having a preexisting condition and how intermittent fasting may interact with this preexisting condition.

For instance, hypoglycemia is a very uncomfortable condition which is triggered by low blood sugar and aggravated during periods of fasting. While it is not generally life-threatening, it can cause a serious reaction in which the sufferer may lose consciousness and become unable to function appropriately.

This is why the first step for newcomers to the intermittent fasting movement is to have a talk with their doctor. This talk can help determine if there is any medical reason why intermittent fasting may not be right for them.

So, let's take a look at some preexisting conditions and how intermittent fasting may affect them.

Diabetes

Diabetics usually need to take medication and follow a rather strict diet in order to keep their condition under control. This includes eating at certain times of the day, restricting sugar and carb consumption while drinking water.

In general, intermittent fasting is not recommended for diabetics though it pays to talk to your doctor and see if some shorter fasting periods may be beneficial to help keep blood sugar down.

On the whole, it may help through the reactions by the body may not be quite as straightforward.

As such, the biggest risk that diabetics may encounter is an imbalance of blood sugar levels. So, a drastic drop in blood sugar may produce dizzy spells and fainting.

Nevertheless, intermittent fasting may be a viable alternative for diabetics to help get their blood sugar in check. Check with your doctor to see if this may be right for you.

Pregnancy and Nursing

While pregnancy is not a preexisting condition as such, intermittent fasting while pregnant and nursing is generally not recommended. This is due to the fact that pregnancy usually has a significant nutritional requirement on the body. Also, a lack of nutrition may adversely affect the baby.

Therefore, it is not recommended during pregnancy, but shorter fasting periods may still yield the same health benefits without harming your child.

As always, check with your doctor if intermittent fasting is right for you.

Digestive Disorders

For folks who have digestive disorders such as Irritable Bowel Syndrome, gastritis, ulcers or colon issues, intermittent fasting may actually be a good option to help relieve these conditions.

Since intermittent fasting forces the digestive system to clear out any residual matter, it offers your digestive system the opportunity to start from scratch, if you will. In addition, your digestive system will take a break, especially if it is overloaded by constant eating. This is important to note as folks who overeat, or eat very frequently, keep their digestive system running at all times.

As such, giving your digestive system a break could be a viable alternative for digestive conditions. While it may not actually heal as such, giving your digestive system a break is certainly beneficial in alleviating many of the conditions we have outlined throughout this book.

Of course, it pays to check with your doctor to see if intermittent fasting will actually aggravate your condition rather than alleviating it. For instance, gastritis sufferers often report pain and discomfort when they go long periods without food. In those cases, the 5:2 method may actually be a very good alternative.

Furthermore, if you are taking medication for any of these conditions, a trip to your doctor's office may keep you from aggravating your condition.

Eating Disorders

One important consideration with intermittent fasting is if a person has a history of eating disorders. For example, conditions such as anorexia and bulimia often involved food deprivation. As such, intermittent fasting may trigger these conditions or even aggravate them in those people who have a history of such conditions.

Therefore, intermittent fasting would be recommended under proper supervision and only if the dieter is medically cleared to attempt this type of eating plan. Since folks recovering from eating disorders often have a long road to recovery, they might show signs of undernourishment months after beginning treatment. Therefore, it pays to discuss this option with your doctor in order to ensure that it is medically safe for the dieter.

Otherwise, the 5:2 method may provide an interesting alternative since it encourages healthy food during fasting periods. Consequently, this method may be implemented under proper medical supervision while ensuring that the dieter receives any support they need in case they show signs of relapsing in their eating disorders.

Final Considerations

Based on the cautions presented in this chapter, it's worth talking to your doctor before engaging in intermittent fasting. In fact, this could be the perfect occasion to work with your doctor and/or nutrition professionals to help you set up a healthy eating plan, especially if you suffer from any type of condition.

While conditions such as digestive distress and diabetes may keep you from getting the medical clearance you need, intermittent fasting may become a viable option for you so that you can achieve the health and fitness goals you have always wanted to achieve, thus ensuring that you can obtain the health benefits we have outlined herein.

Since empirical data shows that folks with a wide range of conditions find improvement through intermittent fasting, it is highly recommended that you check out the possibility of engaging in the dietary practice. At the end of the day, improving your eating habits will only improve your overall quality of life. So, it pays to take a closer look at the options which intermittent fasting can provide you.

Conclusion

If you have made it this far, then you are serious about learning how intermittent fasting can help you become a better version of yourself.

I know that we have covered a lot in this book, but I hope that you now have a good understanding of you can benefit from intermittent fasting by using the methods we have described in this book. I am sure that you are eager to get started, but what's the next step?

I would encourage you to sit down and think about what you really want to get out of this new eating plan.

Are you only looking to lose weight?

Are you looking to drop some pounds and get into better shape?

Do you have a medical condition that requires you to make some lifestyle changes?

Whatever you answer to this question, it's important that you set realistic expectations.

For example, you could choose to set a modest target of dropping one pound per week. Perhaps your goal is to boost your energy or improve your concentration.

Next, think about which method you are going to use.

You could choose to start off with the 5:2 method and build your way up to the 16/8 and eventually up to the Eat-stop-eat method. Or, you could just stick to one method which provides the best results for you.

At the end of the day, you need to choose the method that works best for you. That is the method with which you feel most comfortable.

As you begin to ease your way into the intermittent fasting way of life, you can begin to track the way your body reacts to fasting. You can choose to keep a journal in order to chronicle how your body changes as intermittent fasting becomes a regular part of your life.

It's also important for you to bear in mind that intermittent fasting is not a race. You aren't on the clock. So, there's no rush. You can gradually build up your stamina to a point where you can feel comfortable with the discipline that fasting requires.

Also, try your best to make wholesome lifestyle changes with will boost your fasting efforts. By making significant changes to your lifestyle, you will be able to get the most out of the intermittent fasting way of life.

In fact, I say, "intermittent fasting way of life" because intermittent fasting will eventually become the way that you live your regular, day-to-day life. After all, you are in this for the long haul. You didn't make this decision hoping to achieve incredible results overnight. You decided to embark on this journey knowing that you will have a solid lifestyle plan for the rest of your life.

So, what are you waiting for?

If you have made up your mind, then you can begin by defining what you want out of your new lifestyle. By making gradual and incremental changes to your lifestyle, you can begin to lose weight, feel better about yourself, and turbocharge your body's systems.

So, I would like to thank you for taking the time to read this book. I hope that you have found the information herein useful and informative. If so, then please share it with your friends, family, colleagues, and anyone you feel will be interested in learning more about intermittent fasting. You can become a change agent within your social circle. By sharing this information, you will be helping others become the best they can become.

In addition, don't be afraid to surround yourself with like-minded people. As I have stated earlier, they will help you stay motivated, especially during those days when you are down and wish to give up. They will help you keep your eyes on the prize while you recover your energies and get back in the fight.

I wish you all the best in your endeavor, and do come back any time you need to refresh on any of the contents in this book. By reviewing, you will be able to build on your ideas and experiences.

Thanks again, and good luck.

Description

"Intermittent Fasting: The Complete Beginners Guide to Intermittent Fasting to Rapidly Lose Weight, Burn Fat, and Heal Your Body" Is a book you should read if you are interested in learning more about how you can improve your health, lose weight, boost your self-esteem and, in essence, become the best version of yourself.

This book offers an in-depth look into Intermittent Fasting and its life-changing benefits. The topics it tackles include:

- How to Take the First Step
- Weight Loss
- Causes of Weight Gain and Obesity
- Keeping Your Metabolism on its Toes
- Different Fasting Techniques
- The History of Fasting
- The Best Food Options You Can Take
- And More...